Thomas Faulkner

The Book of Nature

Thomas Faulkner

The Book of Nature

ISBN/EAN: 9783742833600

Manufactured in Europe, USA, Canada, Australia, Japa

Cover: Foto ©Lupo / pixelio.de

Manufactured and distributed by brebook publishing software
(www.brebook.com)

Thomas Faulkner

The Book of Nature

THE

BOOK OF NATURE,

A FULL AND EXPLICIT

EXPLANATION OF ALL THAT CAN OR OUGHT TO BE KNOWN OF THE

STRUCTURE AND USES

OF

The Organs of Life and Generation,

IN

MAN AND WOMAN.

INTENDED ESPECIALLY

FOR

THE MARRIED, OR THOSE INTENDING TO MARRY,

AND WHO CONCIENTIOUSLY AND HONESTLY DESIRE TO INFORM THEM-
SELVES UPON THE INTENT AND NATURE OF

CONJUGAL PLEASURES AND DUTIES.

By THOMAS FAULKNER, M. D.

TO WHICH IS ADDED

A Complete Medical Treatise

UPON ALL

DISEASES OF THE GENERATIVE ORGANS,

WHETHER RESULTING FROM INFECTION OR SEXUAL EXCESSES AND ABUSE.

ILLUSTRATED WITH MORE **THAN FIFTY** ENGRAVINGS

FULLY DEPICTING THE MYSTERIOUS PROCESS OF GESTATION, FROM
THE TIME OF CONCEPTION TO THE PERIOD OF DELIVERY. NO
SUCH COMPLETE PANORAMA OF THE MYSTERIES OF
HUMAN REPRODUCTION HAS EVER BEFORE
BEEN GIVEN TO THE WORLD.

NEW YORK:
HURST & CO., PUBLISHERS,
Nos. 75 & 77 NASSAU STREET.

PREFACE.

"Man, know thyself." It is astonishing that men will dive to the bottom of the deepest seas, and climb to the top of the highest mountains to examine into some secret of Nature, of little if any practical use to any one; while at the same time not the slightest attention is paid to those vital phenomena, upon which rest all of human health and happiness. This is partly owing to the fact that nearly all books that attempt to explain or elucidate the laws of Procreation are either so enveloped in abstruse medical phraseology as to be worse than *Greek* to the general reader, or they are so loosely and broadly treated of as to be unpleasant for the sensitive student.

In this work we have succeeded in avoiding either of these extremes. We have treated in a plain, practical manner the whole wonderful and mysterious matters that properly appertain to the Book of Nature. In opening wide the hitherto sealed pages of this book, we have allowed nothing to escape us that could prove useful and interesting to the student of human formation and procreation. We enter into the arcana of generation; we treat fully and exhaustively of the most important act that man and woman can perform: the creation of beings "but a little lower than the angels." We show both by expressive verbal description and accurate pictorial delineation the various organs and their important uses; we plainly portray the inevitable evils generated by a departure from the true Laws of Nature; and show what pleasing and satisfactory results flow from the proper and legitimate performance of the nuptial rites. We show when, where, and how marriages should be entered into and consummated; we explain how healthy children can be produced, and clearly show how every departure from the laws of nature inevitable entail suffering and disease upon either parents or offspring, and not unfrequently upon both. We show in this book how the married may be as happy as possible, and produce offspring that will in all human probability be healthy and long-lived. We also show the fearful results that follow all unnatural and unhallowed indulgencies, which sap the strength of the body, and bring the intellect to certain and premature decay. Our motive and intent is to do good. To make healthy and happy wives and husbands, daughters and sons.

With this purpose we commend this book to the careful perusal of all who honestly desire to know the whole wonderful mystery of their formation, and procreative desires and faculties.

THE AUTHOR.

THE BOOK OF NATURE.

CHAPTER I.

VEGETABLE REPRODUCTION.

FROM the simplest vegetable to the highest animal we find life displaying its powers, forces and organisms in the most wonderful and beautiful manner; but there is one power in all living things beyond all others wonderful—the power of reproduction. All life on the earth would soon perish if plants and animals of every kind were not provided with the means of producing similar organizations. A tree may live thousands of years, but it perishes at last. There are vegetables and animals that live but a few hours. The individual dies, but the race survives, because the individual is provided with wondrous power of producing other individuals to carry on the life of the race or species. The function of reproduction is therefore of the highest importance and dignity. It is the word of creation for ever going forward. The production of a plant or animal, its development from a living germ, the gradual formation of all its organs, and its whole life processes are very wonderful ; but the most wonderful thing any plant or animal can do is to reproduce itself—to pass on its life in similar organisms, so that its species may be continued for an indefinite period. It is this grandest of the functions of life that we have now to examine.

In the vegetable kingdom, where this phenomenon may be most conveniently examined, there are several modes of reproduction; even the same plant may have two or three distinct methods of propagating its kind. Let us look at our lovely friend of the earliest spring-time, the crocus. Each bulb sends up its flower, and each flower produces germs and pollen. The germ is formed in the ovary or female organ of the flower; the pollen is formed upon the anther, the top of the stamen or male organ. The pollen, a cell containing the masculine element, fertilises the germ-cell, or feminine element, and in some way, incomprehensible to us, the union of the two elements results in the formation of the living germ, which, under favorable circumstances, developes into the perfect plant, which in turn produces new flowers and seeds.

The flower of every plant, and its seed or fruit, is the consummation of its life. On flowers nature has lavished all her ingenuity of construction and adaptation, beauty, perfume, and sweetness. In most plants the masculine and feminine elements are in the same flower, stamens and pistils growing almost in contact. In upright flowers the stamens are longest so that the pollen can fall upon the pistil; in drooping flowers it is the reverse. The snow-drop at first holds up its pure petals to the sun, but when the period comes for the masculine and feminine elements to form the living germs of new beings, it modestly hangs down its head, and it is this change which makes that union possible.

"One analogy," says Flint, " of the world of animal life is still preserved, and the male-flowers as the stronger and bolder sex, are drawn by the impulses of Nature to pay court to the feebler and more delicate female. The male stamina, with their gayly-painted hats, bow around the female pistil as beaux around their belle. Each in turn is permitted to come in contact with the fair, and as the contact takes place, the golden pollen is shaken upon the pistil, and the stamen retires to give place to the next that offers the same hommage. The mystery of fructification is accomplished, and the flower-cup is fecundated.

"There are stamina which can not reach half the height of their beloved pistils. Nature then varies the arrangement, so as not to be defeated in her object. The Lilliputians strive in vain to reach their Brobdignag Venus. As they can not come to her she condescendingly comes down to them. It is in this way that the crown imperial and harebell hang upon their stems, which position, so graceful in the flower, is a foresight of Nature. The pollen of the **stamens comes in contact** with the stigma of the **pistil by** falling upon it. **As soon as the mystery is** accomplished **and the flower-cup** fecundated, the stalk which sustains the flower **turns** it up **toward the sky.** Its bower of love was concealed, but it shows the cradle **of its children.**

"Wherever you see **flowers gently inclining their bells toward** the turf, you may **infer that the stamens within are shorter than** the pistil. There **are** plants, **the habits of whose loves are still** more amusing. They are the wedded dames who in compassion to their little husbands, slightly bend their elastic persons, contemplate them for a moment, and afterward erect themselves, still bearing marks of their yielding weakness. Such are the **loves of the passion-flower and the willow-herb."**

Many flowers are provided with organs which secrete honey; this honey is stored in deep vases, very deep sometimes, as in the Columbine Bees and other insects, and even some birds, as the humming bird, attracted by the honey, and seeking it in its deep cells, unconsciously aid in the process of generation. The pollen adheres to **their bodies or wings, and is** brought in contact with the stigma of **the** same flower, **or others** of the **same species, to which** they are made to adhere by a viscid **secretion. All flowers do not contain** both male and female organs of generation. They may be on different parts of the same plant, as in the maize, or corn, where the pollen is produced **on** the very top of the tall stalk, sometimes twenty feet **high, while the long** silky pistils grow from the cob which holds the **germs in rows** about the middle of the stalk. **Sometimes** the **male and female flowers are** on different trees or plants, and **their propagation is entirely dependent upon insect or favoring** breezes.

When the pollen **cell,** containing the fecundating element falls upon the stigma of a flower, adhering to its viscid secretion, a very beautiful vital process commences. The inner membrane of the pollen extends itself into a tube which penetrates into **the** style, which is sometimes two or three inches in length, until it reaches the **germ in the ovary, where it** penetrates **the germ, or meets a corresponding tube thrown out by it.** The **two elements unite, the germ is** fertilised and **grows into a seed, the egg of** the plant, **in which is formed, and from** which **is de**veloped the new plant **which is to continue the** species. The living **germ of the plant is** very **small, quite microscopic in its dimensions.** The **seeds of plants contain albuminous and oily matter, destined to be the first food of the young plant, and which also, in such seeds as those of wheat, barley, rice, peas, beans, &c., furnish important stores of food for men and animals.** If **we examine** such seeds, we shall find **the** real germ to be a mere speck, a microscopic cell, which must, however, contain potentially the future plant or **tree, and all** it is capable of **producing; must contain form, character, color, odor, and the**

Fig. 1.

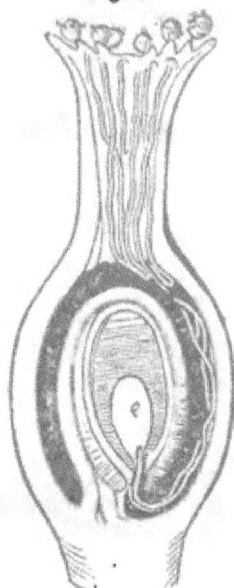

SECTION OF PISTIL, with Pollen Grains, sending tubes down to the ovary.

directive or formative principle which governs its whole life and development. And this character of the plant, observe, resides in the two elements, **male and female,** which join **to produce it, for** by bringing together **these** elements, gardeners are **able to** produce all kinds of crosses, hybrids, and **varieties.**

The reproduction or continuation of **the species of plants by this process is called true generation; but this is not the only mode by which vegetable life is continued** or extended. **The bulb** of our crocus which **sends up a stalk,** leaves, and flower also throws out from its side fibres which form new bulbs, which the following season separate from the parent bulb, and themselves produce **bulbs and flowers.**

Take now a tuberous plant—the potato. It has its pretty flowers, and produces balls full of seeds which will produce new plants and varieties; but at the same time there grow out from the roots great tubers, and on these are buds which will grow into perfect plants, producing in turn seeds and tubers. The straw_ berry has also a double method of propagation. It produces flowers and seeds, but it also throws out long vines, which at intervals send down roots on which grow plants, and so on until a whole field is covered with them.

We imitate these processes of nature in multiplying plants and trees—of one making many. Ladies cut slips of geraniums, roses and other plants, placing them in pots of moist sand or earth when the covered buds send out roots, and those exposed to the light expand into leaves. The Chinese multiply fruit trees by moulding a ball of earth upon a twig, keeping it moist, and making a section in the bark below it. When roots have penetrated the earth they cut it off and plant it. Each bud of a tree has its distinct life, and in most cases can be transferred to another tree of an allied species and made to grow, producing, however, its own peculiar flowers and fruit. Each bud is a germ; the seed germs are similar, but differ at least in this, that they sometimes produce as in potatoes and apples, new varieties. A bud or graft gives us the same fruit as its parent tree. A tree which grows from an apple seed may produce very different fruit. For this reason, when fruit trees are grown from seeds, gardeners bud or graft them; that is, transfer to them buds or twigs from trees producing a favorite variety, and let the transferred buds grow to form the future trees.

Low forms of vegetation, as the various kinds of fungi and ferns are produced from spores, which are germs or rudimental buds rather than seeds. They are very small, produced by myriads, as in the puff ball, and are so light as to be blown about by the winds, and almost fill the atmosphere. Wherever air can penetrate, it carries with it the germs of vegetation as well as those of the lower forms of animal life.

But it is in our lovely and odorous flowers that we have the highest types of the generation of vegetable life; and the favorite science of Botany largely consists of the study of the organs and processes of vegetable reproduction, or what the Elder Darwin in his curious poem calls the Loves of the Plants, which present us with the most delightful analogies to the higher processes of reproduction in animals and our own species. Botany is therefore a charming introduction to all other branches of natural history, and especially to that branch of human physiology which we are now considering.

CHAPTER II.

ANIMAL REPRODUCTION.—THE ORIGIN OF LIFE.

REPRODUCTION in animals is curiously analogous to the same process in the vegetable kingdom. There are the same varieties in the modes of multiplication and generation. The process of generation in some of the lower animal organizations is exactly like the throwing out of new bulbs in plants. The polypes throw out buds which in a little while grow mouths, fringed with cilia or tentacles, while they are still holding by stalks, and drawing part of their nourishment from their parents. When enough matured to get their own living they drop off, swim away, and shift for themselves. This is gemmation.

Fission is a common mode of propagation or multiplication among the infusoria. An animalcule is seen to contract in a ring around its centre; the fissure deepens, and it divides into two distinct beings, which also divide, and so on—multiplying with surprising rapidity. It has been estimated that one of these animalcules could produce by these successive divisions in eight weeks a progeny of two hundred and sixty-eight millions. This reproductive power is, however, almost rivalled by some fishes and insects. The carp lays seven hundred thousand eggs in a season, and lives two hundred years. The possible progeny of a pair of these fishes is almost beyond computation. The cod is said to produce from four to nine millions of eggs. The female termite lays sixty thousand eggs a day for a considerable period.

Some of the lower animals may be multiplied artificially like vegetables. Thus, if some species of the polypus are cut in pieces, each piece produces the missing parts, so as to become a perfect animal, as cuttings of a geranium produce geraniums.

But perhaps the most curious mode of multiplication takes place in some sea-worms. They divide into sections by constricting rings, and its section forms for itself head, eyes, &c., at one extremity, and tail at the other, while yet the sections are united; but when all is ready each section sets up its own independent life, and then produces in its body germs of similar worms, by the more usual process—just as some vegetables propagate by seeds, as well as by bulbs or tubers.

These modes of multiplication—fission, gemmation, &c., such as I have described are, however, not the rule in nature, but the exception, or variation—a ruder method of the extension of life, which is confined to the lower forms of animal existence. As vegetables are generally produced from seeds, animals are generally produced from eggs.

It has long been a disputed question with the learned, as to whether life can be produced, under certain circumstances from inanimate substances, independent of egg or seed, without parental scource. Numerous experiments have been tried to solve this problem, and some have seemed to determine the question affirmatively, but more searching investigation has detected the fallacy of the experiments, and at present the majority of Physiologists disbelieve the doctrine of spontaneous generation.

There is no good reason, so far as we now know, to believe that there is any spontaneous generation of vegetables or animals— that is, that any vegetable or animal ever of itself is formed from matter without a spore or germ which has been produced by a similar organization. At some time, and in some way, every kind of living form has its beginning; but no one has seen such beginning. Creation is a mystery. Every living thing upon the earth has at some time, somewhere and somehow been created; but we do not know the when, the where, or the how. Human science reveals to us something of the phenomena of nature— nothing of its causes or beginnings.

As in vegetables we find the beginning of new organizations in the formation by the generative organs of a plant, which are in most cases portions of its flower, of a germ cell in the ovary or female organ, and of a pollen cell by the anthor or male organ, which unite to form the living germ, which develops into the perfect plant—so in all the higher forms of animal life, in oysters, fishes, insects, birds, beasts, and men, we have germs or eggs formed in the ovaries of the female, which at a certain stage of development are impregnated, or fecundated by union with a similar germ, produced in a somewhat similar organ of the male —the male and female elements uniting to produce the perfect being. The unfertilised, unimpregnated, or unfecundated ovum or egg quickly perishes. The one to which has been added the masculine element is from that moment endowed with life, and, with favoring conditions, developes with a wonderful rapidity.

Fishes produce a vast number of eggs, as may be seen in the hard roe of herring, which, when they have arrived at a certain stage, are spawned—that is, expelled from the body in places which the fish instinctively find for that purpose. Salmon come hundreds, perhaps thousands of miles, through the deep ocean to lay their eggs in the shallow fresh water streams in which they themselves were hatched. The male herring and salmon produce, in organs not unlike the ovaries, myriads of sperm cells, destined to fertilise the germ cells of the female. This is the soft roe—a brain-like substance, chiefly composed of these cells. The male fishes attend the females, and fill the water where their eggs are laid with what seems a milky fluid. The two elements come into contact, perhaps by a mutual attraction, fecundation takes place, and, in due time, swarms of young fishes are the result.

With insects and birds, the process is a little varied. The eggs are formed, as with the fishes, in the ovaries of the females, but at a certain stage they are fecundated before leaving the body, by the male element being conveyed to them by a process similar to that which takes place in flowers. The seminal fluid of the male, corresponding to the pollen of the plant, is conveyed to the germ in the ovary by means specially adapted to that purpose. After the egg has grown to its full size—in insects covered with a tough membrane, and in birds with a hard shell—it is placed in some proper nest, and hatched either by solar heat or the warmth of one or both of the parents. Animals so born are called oviparous—born from eggs. A few fishes, as the shark and skate, lay fecundated eggs like birds, with curiously formed horny shells, and cables for mooring.

With the mammalia, the higher orders of animals, including the human species, there is still another process. The egg or germ is formed in the ovary of the female. When fully formed it bursts from its containing membranes, with a certain degree of excitement of the generative system, and passes through tubes provided for that purpose into a receptacle called the uterus, or womb. If here met by the seminal fluid, or fertilising masculine element, fecundation takes place, a perfect germ is produced, foetal life begins, and the animal is, so to speak, hatched in the womb of its mother, nourished by her blood, and grows until it is ready to come into the world and live its independent life. Animals so produced are called viviparous, or born alive.

The young of the kangaroo, and other marsupials, are born in a very immature condition, and carried in a kind of bag formed upon the abdomen of the mother ; within which are the teats from which the little ones draw their nourishment.

The eggs of birds, from those of the humming-bird, like peas, to the great eggs of the ostrich, which will furnish a dinner for six men, contain not only the germ, which is very minute, but its supply of food—the materials from which its body bones, feathers, &c., are formed, during the process of incubation or hatching. The white of the egg, almost pure albumen, is not essential to it, but useful as food. The eggs of many animals are without it. The yolk, consisting of albumen and oil, contains tho matter first taken into the organization. The germinal spot, a point of matter, is the real germ, and can only bo seen under the microscope. The eggs of viviparous animals are of extreme minuteness. That of a dog is the 1-130th of an inch in diameter including yolk, germinal vesicle, and germinal spot. The human ovum is still smaller, about 1-140th of an inch in diameter ; and in the circumference of that small diameter lies, what a world of character and power !—lies all that shall distinguish the highest example of human civilization and culture, from the lowest savage—poet, philosopher, hero, idiot, ruffian, lunatic—all the possibilities and potentialities of humanity.

CHAPTER III.

THE ORGANS OF GENEBATION.

In the human race, as throughout the greater part of the animal kingdom, generation is accomplished by fecundation, or the effect of the vivifying fluid provided by one class of organs upon the germ contained in the seed or ovum formed by another class, in the opposite sex. This germ, when fecundated, is termed the embryo. The process consists of impregnation in the male—conception in the female.

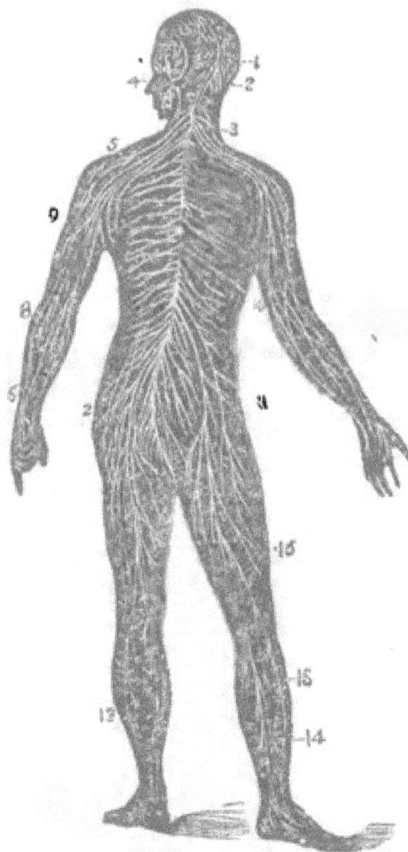

The organs of generation in the male are—1. The testes and their envelopes, namely, the scrotum or cutaneous envelope: the dartos, which corrugates or ridges the scrotum; and the fibrous or vaginal tunics ; we must also here include the epidermis, above the testes; the vas deferens, or excretory duct, and the spermatic chord. 2. Vesiculæ seminales, forming a canal situated beneath the bladder. 3. The prostate gland, surrounding the neck of the bladder and the commencement of the urethra. 4. Cowper's glands, a pair situated below the prostate. 5. The ejaculatory ducts. 6. The penis, which consists of the corpus cavernosum, the urethra, the corpus spongiosum, which terminates in the glans penis: then there are the vessels, nerves, and a cutano-

THE NERVOUS SYSTEM.

1. The cerebrum; 2. cerebellum; 3, spinal cord; 4, nerves of the face; 5, the bracial plexus or union of nerves; 6, 7. 8, 9, nerves of the arm; 10, those that pass under the ribs; 11. lumbar plexus; 12. sacral plexus; 13, 14, 15, 16, nerves of the lower limbs.

ous investment, which by its prolongation forms the prepuce.

The female organs are: 1. The vulva or pupendum, the external parts, comprehending the labia pupendi, the clitoris, situated at the middle and supperior part of the pupendum; the nymphæ or alæ minores; the urethra, which terminates in the meatus urinarius, opening into the vagina, which is occupied by the hymen, a semilunar fold or the carunculæ myrtiformis, its lacerated remains, and the entrance into the vagina, termed the os externum, so called to distinguish it from the internum, or orifice of— 2. The uterus, whose appendages are—the ligamenta lata (the broad ligaments). sometimes called alæ vespertilionum, and the round ligaments commencing immediately before and below the Fallopian tubes, which extend to the ovaria.

THE PERINÆUM.—The space between the anus and the external parts of the generative organs, so called from being frequently moist. The operation of cutting for stone in males is usually performed here.

The Bladder is the receptacle for the urine, which it receives by drops from the *Ureters*, the conduits from the kidneys. In shape the bladder is somewhat like a pear; but it is much modified by the quantity of its contents, and the relative condition of the neighboring parts. For instance, when the bladder is full, its upper part may be distinguished as rising above the *Pubes*, or that portion of the lower part of the abdomen that is covered with hair. The bladder is composed of several coats. There is a peculiar membrane investing the important structures in the abdomen called the *peritonœum*. The fundus and back part of the bladder is covered by a portion of this peritonœum, which serves in some measure to support the bladder in its position.

Fig. 3.

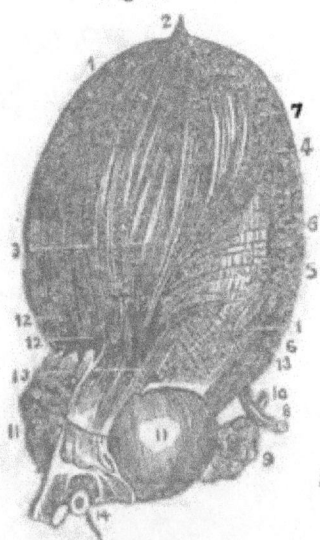

URINARY BLADDER shawing its muscular fibres. 8 Left Ureter. 9 Left portion of Seminal Vesicles. 11, 11. Lateral lobes of the Prostate Gland. 14 Uretra tied with a cord.

The muscular coats of the bladder are very strong; they consist of fibres running in three different directions. An idea of their strength may be given, when it is stated, that the bladder is capable of containing *per force, two or three pints of urine,* the whole of which can be ejected to the last drop.

The ureters open very obliquely into the bladder, for the two-fold purpose of preventing a retrogression of the urine, and its too rapid descent into the bladder. The bladder, as the urine accumulates in it, becomes sensibly excited to contraction · and hence the discarge.

The Kidneys, which appear to form so insignificant an item in the human body, are among the most important structures in its economy. By some wonderful, yet inexplicable process, the waste fluid of the body, except that given off by perspiration and exhalation, passes through them. All we know of the matter is, that the blood in its circulation wends its way through especial arteries called the Renal, and comes out through the ureters in the form

Fig. 4.

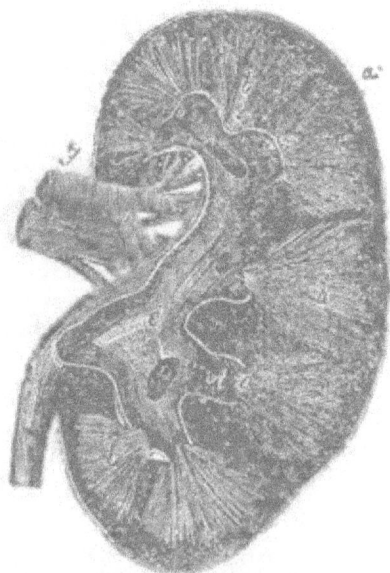

of urine, the rapidity of which process, in some instances, is most astonishing. Diseases of the kidneys form a serious malady, and often jeopardize the life of man. The kidneys will be perceived to be situated in the upper part of the loins.

The kidneys are usually embedded in fat. The exterior coat of the kidney is very vascular, and the inner consists of tubes collected into conical points that open into the pelvis of the kidney.

Section of a Kidney.

CHAPTER IV.

GERMINATION, FECUNDATION AND IMPREGNATION.

At a certain period in the life of a plant, in organs prepared for that important function, are formed the germs of new plants. The germ-producing organ, frond or flower, does its work and dies. The tree lives on, but each individual bud, producing flower and seed or fruit perishes. This is the law of vegetative generation. Such is also, to a great extent, the law of insect life.

Fig. 5.

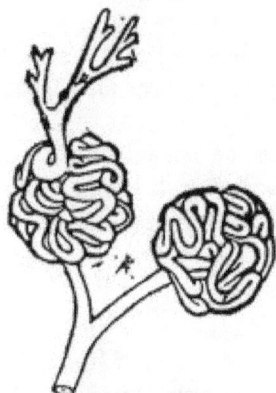

Or Malpigian bodies, from the kidney of an owl, injected and very largely magnified. These bodies as well as the testes, offer fine examples of the extension of secreting surface by the convolution of tubes.

Renal Glands.

Fig. 7.

Fig 6.

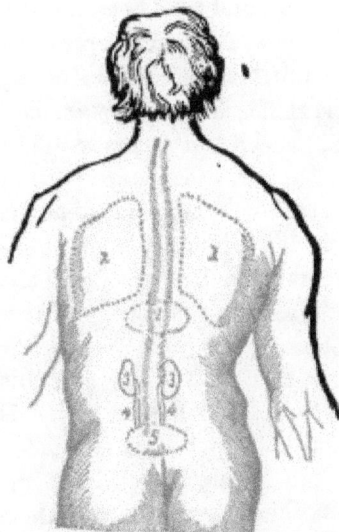

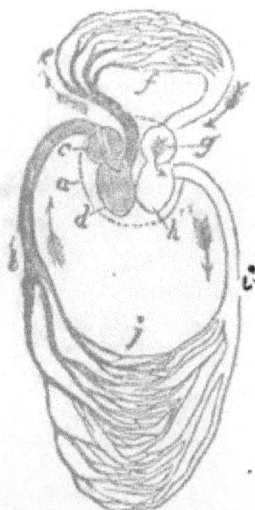

BACK VIEW OF THE BODY.

1, 1, The Lungs; 2, the Stomach; 3; 3, the Kidneys; 4, 4, the Ureters; 5, the Bladder.

IDEAL VIEW OF THE COURSE OF CIRCULATION.

a, Encloses the four chambers of the heart; b, Veins bringing dark blood to c, right auricle ; d, right ventricle ; e, pulmonary artery ; f, Beginning of pulmonary vein conveying the arterialized blood to g, left auricle; h, left ventricle; i arteries. The arrows show the directions of the current.

The insect produces one crop of germs ; they are fertilized by
one conjunction of the sexes ; the eggs are deposited, sometimes
in immense numbers, where they can be hatched in safety, and
where its proper food can be found for the new being in the
earliest stage of its development; and then, as if the whole purpose of life had been accomplished, the male and female alike
perish.   In some cases the male insect sacrifices his life in the
very act of fecundation.

In the higher orders of, animals, fishes, reptiles, birds, and
mammals, the production of germs goes on year after year in·
varying periods.   The guinea pig begins to breed at two months
old, and the higher the type, the later is the period of germ formation, until in man the period of puberty, or the beginning of
the generative function, is at about fifteen years, varying from
twelve to eighteen; but the natural powers are scarcely at their
full strength and fitness until some years later.

The power of reproduction as to numbers seems to be in the
inverse ratio as to development.   The lowest forms of life multiply
with amazing rapidity; some insects produce myriads, fishes
spawn eggs by millions, hens lay an egg a-day for months together,
rabbits, cats, dogs breed every few months, and have at each birth
a numerous progeny, while the higher orders of mammalia produce
their young but once a-year, and have but òne, or, in rare cases,
two at a birth.   When the human germ has been slowly formed
in the ovary, and perfected up to the period when it bursts forth
in its first birth, fit for impregnation, it is nine months in arriving
at the development which fits it for birth and independent
existence.   For twelve months more it draws its supply of nutri-
ment from the mother, and two years may be considered the
normal interval from birth to birth.   It should never be less with
a proper regard to the health of the mother, and the proper
development of her children; and the practice of shortening this
period by hiring wet nurses is a violation of nature which is
avenged on parents and their offspring.   The mother is exhausted
by too frequent child bearing, and children are deprived of the
love, the magnetism, the life of the mother, which comes to them
from her blood transformed into the most delicious food for them,
and the nervous and spiritual food which no money can buy, and
no one but the mother can give.

The human germ cell, or egg, is formed from the blood in a gland-like organ, about an inch and a-half long, oval shaped placed in the lower part of the abdomen, in the groin, and situated on each side of the uterus, or womb (Fig. 15). In each ovary, from the period of puberty, in a healthy female, there is a constant formation and growth of germs, or ova, which goes on for thirty or forty years. When the first perfect germs have ripened, one or more, they come to the surface of the ovary, burst from their sacs, sometimes with considerable force, attended by a nervous excitement, a congestion of the blood vessels of ovaries and womb, and, when impregnation does not take place, the freed germ passes into the mouth of the Fallopian tube, through which it passes into the uterus from which it passes, with the menstrual evacuation, a secretion from the mucous surfaces of these organs, reddened more or less by some exudation from the congested vessels, through the mouth of the womb into the vagina. This menstrual, or monthly flow, marking the production of germs, and their expulsion when not fecundated by the presence of the masculine element, goes on monthly, from its commencement at the age of puberty, normally at fourteen to sixteen years of age,

Fig. 8.

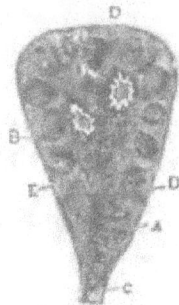

TRANSVERSE SECTION THROUGH THE OVARY.— From a case in the fifth month of pregnancy. a. b. ovisacs. c. ovarian ligament. d d, tunica albuginea. e, stroma. In the interior can be seen two old corpora lutea.

to the period of the cessation of the menses, or "turn of life," from forty-five to sixty, when no more germs are formed, and the capacity for child-bearing ceases.

Corresponding to the ovaries or egg-forming organs of the female, are two similar glandular bodies, called the testes, in the male, which produce the spermatic or seminal fluid, corresponding to the pollen of plants, by which the germs are fertilized, or fecundated ; by means of these germ cells and sperm cells the masculine and feminine elements are brought together so that they can unite in the body and soul, the material and spiritual life of a new being.

The testes, or testicles show the importance of their function by a wonderfully elaborate organization, of which some idea is given in Fig. 5 ; though a very imperfect one, in an ideal section intended to give an outline of the structure. The oval body is composed of a vast number of lobules, formed of very fine tubes closely folded, and everywhere in contact with blood vessels and nerves. There are in each testicle about four hundred and fifty of these lobules. The matter secreted from them passes through a vast number of tubes, 1-170th of an inch in diameter, ending in a convoluted tubular structure measuring twenty-one feet in length, ending in a single tube, which carries the masculine generative matter to the urethra, whence, in the sexual congress, it is ejected into the vagina, enters the mouth of the womb, and either there or in the Fallopian tubes, meets and impregnates the germ coming from the ovaries.

The seminal fluid is as complex and vital a substance as we should expect to have formed by so remarkable an apparatus. Floating in a liquid are minute cells, in which other cells, or corpuscles may be discovered, and in these are formed, as shown in Fig. 18, bundles of spermatozoa, curiously shaped living cells, 1-600 to 1-800 of a line in length, each one of which is furnished with a single cilium, or long slender tail, which propels it with a constant vibrative motion, as if it were a living animalcule. This spermatozoon is believed to be the true agent of fertilization, corresponding to the pollen grain of the flower. It has been discovered in the womb, in the Fallopian tubes, and in contact with the germ just leaving the ovary. There can be little doubt that the cells, furnished with long propellers, as shown in Fig. 17, carry in them the male principle which gives to the female germ all that makes the child resemble its father, all that it inherits from him of bodily form, features, complexion,

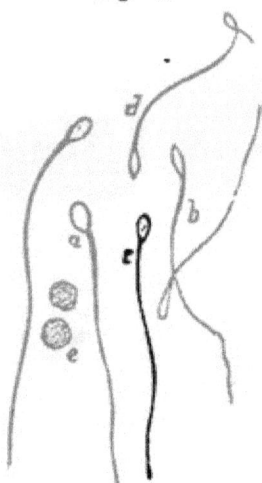

Fig. 9.

HUMAN SPERMATOZOA.

These are magnified from nine hundred to one thousand diameters, a. Spermatozoon presenting the flat surface. b. One viewed in profile. c. Showing a circular spot on the surface, which some suppose to be a sucker. d. Shows an elongation from the head, like a proboscis. e. Granules, or cells, in which other zoosperms are preparing.

temperament, constitution, mental power, and moral character—

health, disease, idiosyncrasy; that which may make his happiness or misery in this life—and who can say how much also in the life to come?

The germs of human, as of all life, are produced in immense numbers. Even in childhood imperfect germs are formed and discharged, and conception may take place before menstruation begins. Idleness, luxury, the use of rich, highly seasoned food, condiments, and stimulants, and the excitement of the passions hasten puberty, and exaggerate and disorder the corresponding masculine function.

The microscope does not reveal to us what takes place in the act of impregnation or conception, or what change is produced by the contact of the spermatozoon with the ovum. The egg of the maiden hen contains the rudiments of the chick, but it can never be hatched. The warmth that brings life and development to the impregnated egg, only hastens the putrifaction of the un-impregnated. The unimpregnated eggs of the frog quickly putrify; but if the male element be soon brought to them they expand into living creatures. In this case the spermatozoa can be seen become embedded in the gelatinous covering of the eggs, they pass through the membranes which cover them, and are probably absorbed into the ovum.

The blood goes to the testes in long, slender, tortuous arteries, presenting an extensive surface for the action of nervous energy, and there is no doubt that the best blood of the body is selected to form the semen, and that it is changed and perfected, first in these arteries and then in the wonderfully fine and convoluted tubes of the testes. The same arteries that supply blood to the testes in the male, furnish the circulation of the ovaries in the female; and the same nervous centres furnish the nerve energy and directing intelligence; but what makes the difference in action—forming germ cells in one sex, and sperm cells in the other—or what makes sex, must probably remain among life's inscrutable mysteries. "Arrest of development" will not account for it, and if it did, what causes arrest of development? "Male and female created He them."

At the age of puberty remarkable changes take place in both sexes. Boys and girls differ indeed from their tenderest years. As a rule boys are more boisterous, girls more gentle; while the girl chooses a doll for her plaything, the boy prefers a drum, a sword, or whip. But at puberty the sexual instincts become stronger, and there is in each a more pronounced development of masculine or feminine appearances and qualities. In the boy the voice deepens in tone, and the face begins to be covered with a beard. Where the testes have been removed, destroyed, or imperfectly developed, the voice remains treble, and the beard light or wanting. There is an enlargement of the throat, the "Adam's apple" corresponding to the full development of the masculine organs. On the other hand the girl becomes at puberty more decidedly feminine, by the enlargement of the pelvis, the broadening of the hips, and the development of the mammary or milk-forming glands in the bosom. There is no beard to mar the delicacy and feminine beauty of the face, but in both sexes alike, at this period, hair appears upon the pubes. The most striking difference, however, is that already mentioned—the occurrence of the monthly period, marking the ripening and expulsion of germs capable of becoming living men and women.

Fig. 10.

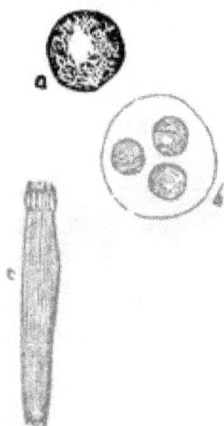

EVOLUTIONS OF ZOOSPERMS.
Objects in human semen, magnified one thousand times. *a.* A large, rounded corpuscle. *b.* A globule of evolution, which incloses three roundish granular bodies. *c.* A bundle of seminal animalcules, as they grouped together in the testicle.

Woman differs from man in her entire organization—mental, emotional, physical. She is more rounded, graceful, soft, sensitive, mobile. Her nervous system is finer and more delicate; she has quicker sensibilities and finer powers of instinct and intuition. Even the bony skeleton of a woman can be distinguished at a glance from that of a man by its longer head and broader pelvis, and generally by its smaller hands and feet. Riche-

Fig. 11.

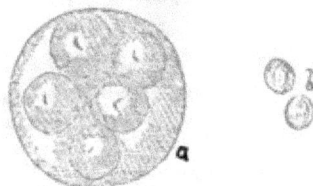

CYST OF EVOLUTION.
This figure is a remarkable view of a seminal cyst, or cell. *a.* Containing five smaller cells, in each of which may be perceived a nucleus. *b.* Two seminal granules; all highly magnified.

rand has, perhaps, exaggerated in saying that "the reproduction of the species is, in woman, the most important object in life—almost the only destination to which nature has called her, and the only duty she has to fulfil in human society;" but Madame de Stael went nearly as far in saying, "Love is but an episode in the life of man; it is the whole history of the life of woman." Byron has said almost in the same words,

"Love is of man's life a thing apart;
'Tis woman's whole existence."

I think, however, that there are women who have brains as well as ovaries; and that even the faculties which make women most charming as wives and most excellent as mothers, may have a much broader scope than the production, care, and education of their own offspring. Hundreds of women who have never borne children have been more than mothers to great multitudes. In the actual condition of humanity there may be a higher work for many woman in saving the children of others, than in having children of their own.

CHAPTER V.

EMBRYOLOGY.

In all nature we find one singular, universal fact. All animals, without exception, high or low, of whatever ultimate complexity or simplicity of structure, originate from eggs, and from eggs of the same character. Some animals, as corals for instance, many hydroids, and other low organisms, reproduce themselves by budding or by division of the parent stock. But they also, at some time or other produce eggs, and thus bear their testimony to the general law of nature which applies to the whole animal kingdom, without exception. Indeed, the seed in plants has the same structure as the so-called ovarian egg in animals, and thus we may speak of all organized

Fig. 12.

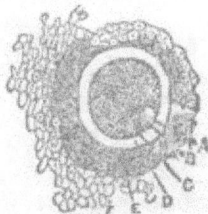

AN OVUM.
a. Germinal spot. b. Germinal vesicle. c. Yolk. d. Zona pellucida. e. discus proligerus. f. adherent granules or cells.

beings, vegetable or animal, as multiplying by eggs. The ovarian egg is microscopic, in many animals, but whatever its size it consists of an outer bag filled with a semi-transparent fluid which is somewhat oily, and an inner bag also filled with a transparent fluid, which is chiefly albuminous. The difference in the character of the two fluids gives greater translucence to that which fills the inner sac. Within the inner bag there is a spot or dot, sometimes several of them, more or less distinct. In this condition, all eggs borne of whatever living creature, are alike.

Fig. 13.

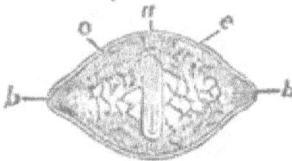

MAMMAL OVUM.

A view of the ovum of a bitch, twenty-three days from the last access of the male. The chorion c. c, has already shot forth little villi, which, however, are wanting at either end, b, b. of the ovum and also over the place where the embryo is situated. This engraving represents its object of the natural size.

All eggs arise in what are called ovaries. These are clusters of cells, forming bunches of a somewhat glandular character in appearance Between these cells the eggs are formed and in such a way as at first to be hardly distinguished from the cells themselves. The same is true of sperm cells, which arise in organs of the same character as the ovary, and are formed in a manner perfectly similar to that of the formation of the egg. So we have these two spheres of growth which characterize sex in the animal kingdom, arising in conditions so very similar that the essence of the two is hardly to be determined by observation.

Fig. 14.

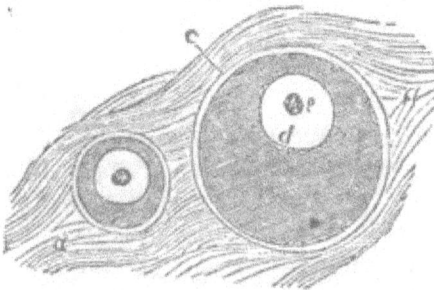

OVA IN THE OVARY.

A magnified view of two eggs of a bird, as they are found in the ovary. They are scarcely perceptible to the naked eye. a, Stroma, or substance of the ovary, composed of thick fibres. c, Chorion, or external membrane of the ovum. b, Yolk. d, Germinal vesicle. e, Germinal spot, which is the real germ from which the embryo is evolved.

In order to fully appreciate what eggs are, we must remember that all organized bodies are composed of little bags which are called cells, and which are formed and multiplied in various ways.

Most of these cells are so small that they can only be perceived by the aid of high magnifying powers. There are, it is true, a few cell structures large enough to be seen with the naked eye, as, for instance, the cell of common elder pith, or the coarse cells of the orange. It is one of the great problems of modern research to ascertain how the different kinds of these cells are

Fig. 15.   Fig. 16.

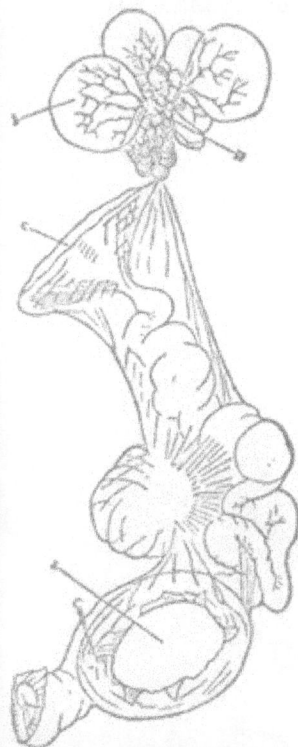

Ovary and Oviduct from a Laying Hen.
a, Immature ovarian eggs. b, Mature ovarian eggs. c. Opening of oviduct which receives the egg when it drops from the ovary. d, Egg with shell, in the lower part of oviduct.

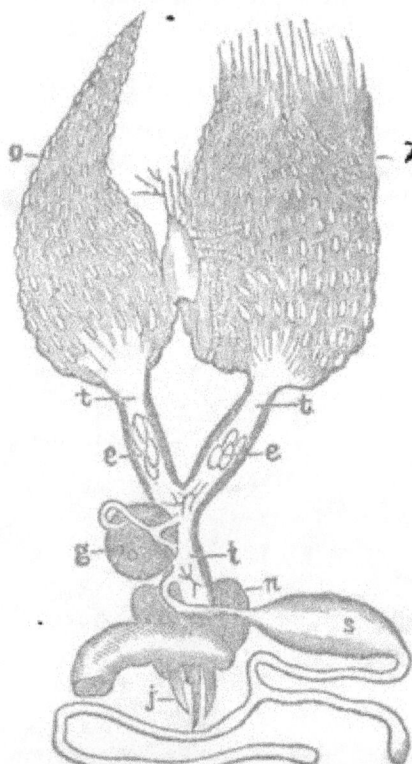

Ovaries, etc., of the Bee.
o, o, Ovaries. t, t, t, Oviducts. e, e, e, Eggs in oviducts. g, Receptaculum seminis. n, j. Sting. s, Poison bag.

formed and what is their mode of reproduction. Some naturalists assume that in the animal substance secreted by a living body, such as milk which is secreted by the mammary glands or similar

substances secreted by other organs, certain particles become
centres of action, around which other particles crowd ; and
when a little collection of this kind, microscopically small,
has been formed, an envelope arises around it, and we have the
utricle or cell. Others believe that minute, imperceptible parti:
cles of animal substance swell and enlarge, and become hollow,
so that a little bag is formed, a cell envelope in short, which fills
as it enlarges with a fluid substance.   There are those, also, who
assume that the two modes of cell formation exist simultaneously
in the same being.

When the ovarian egg has acquired its ultimate growth, prior
to the formation of the germ, the egg of the mammalia presents
a bag, the so-called *zona pellucida*, the walls of which are exceedingly transparent. This bag is filled with a substance which is

Fig. 17.

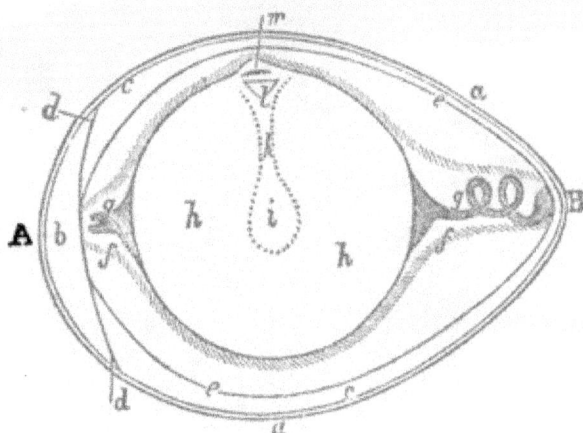

IDEAL SECTION OF A HEN'S EGG.

The egg of the fowl is the type of all ova, and from its large size, is easy
to study. A. Blunt pole. B. Sharp pole. *a, a.* Shell. *b.* Space filled with
air, to supply oxygen. *c.* Membrane of the shell, which, at *d, d,* splits into
two layers. *c, c.* Limits of the second and thicker albumen. *f.* Limits of the
third and thickest albumen, the white being in three layers. *g g.* Chalaze,
or ropes of twisted fibers from the yolk, which hold it in its place. *h.* Yolk.
i. Central cavity in the yolk, from which a duct, *k,* leads to the cicatricula, or
tread. *l.* Cumulous proligerous, or germinal cumulus. *m.* Germ or blastos.
The egg is so formed that the yolk floats high in the white, and the germ is
always uppermost.

itself transparent, and yet which appears, under a very high
magnifying power, to be granular, as if dotted with particles
floating in the fluid. In that outer bag is another diminutive bag

containing also a transparent fluid. This inner bag occupies an eccentric position with reference to the periphery of the outer bag, and in it are contained one or several dots. The outer envelope is called the vitelline membrane, because it corresponds exactly to the exceedingly thin skin inclosing the yolk in the hen's egg. The yolk is called vitellus, and hence the name. The bag contains the yolk, and however transparent this fluid may be, retains the name of yolk. The inner bag is called the germinative vesicle. The dot or dots within the germinative vesicle are ordinarily called the germinative dot or dots.

Fig. 18.

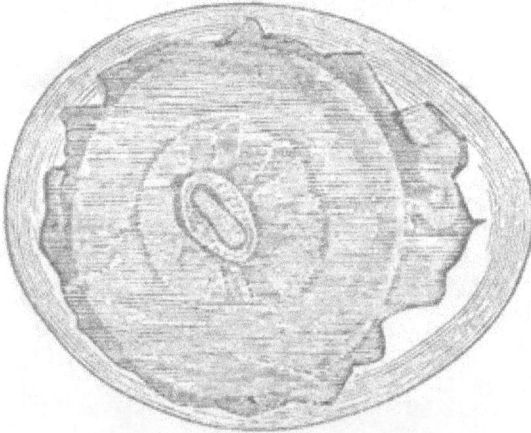

EGG 36 HOURS AFTER INCUBATION.

The dimensions of the mammalian egg are very small. It comes just within the range of the power of the human eye. Place the ovary under the microscope and you will find that it contains eggs of various dimensions in various stages of growth. In some the amount of yolk is less than in others; in some the germinative vesicle and the germinative dot exist; in others they are not yet formed; indeed, vesicles are found in the ovary in which neither germinative dot nor germinative vesicle exists, and which are supposed to be eggs in process of formation.

If we pass now to the bird, we find in the ovary eggs which can in no way be distinguished from those observed in the ovary of the mammal, except that we find in the former a much larger number of them, and their outer envelope is much thinner. Besides those very small ovarian eggs, there are larger ones—eggs rising to dimensions so considerable that they are not only visible to the naked eye, but may be handled with facility. A mature egg in the ovary of the hen is about the dimension of a small walnut. It has no shell, no white; but it is a bulk of yolk inclosed in a vitelline membrane, containing a germinative vesicle with germinative dots. The amount of yolk is very great.

If an ovarian egg of the hen was enlarged so that the germinative vesicle alone would appear as large as a whole ovarian egg at the time of maturity; we should find that the whole of the yolk consists either in little granules or in little vesicles resembling each other so much as almost to force us to the conclusion that these vesicles are only granules which have swollen and become

Fig. 19.

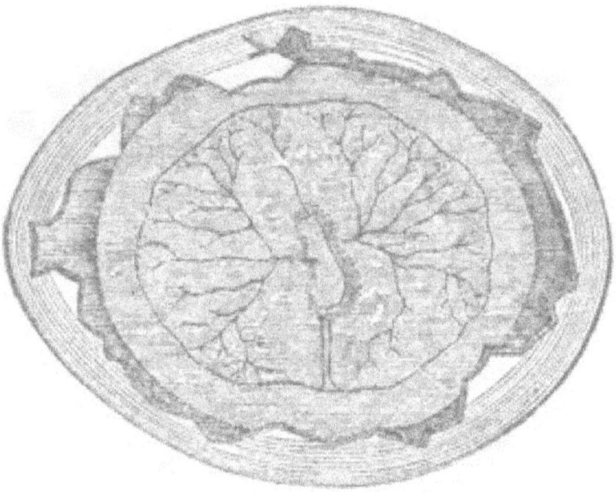

EGG OPENED THREE DAYS AFTER INCUBATION.

hollow. By the side of these smaller vesicles are others somewhat larger, containing themselves a vesicle and granule ; that is to say, having the true character of ordinary cells. The whole mass of the yolk consists of such granular vesicles and true cells. The yolk is, in fact, an accumulation of cells in various stages of growth. A large yolk, or the large ovarian egg of a hen, with its contents, was itself at one time so small as to escape the natural power of the human eye. We may place a portion of the ovary of the hen under the microscope and have at the same time in the field small eggs which cannot be seen with the naked eye, and other eggs perceptible in different degrees ; and we find that the smallest are just like the eggs of mammalia, containing a transparent fluid with granules floating in it, while others contain cells already to be distinguished ; and others are full of cells so large as to make the whole mass opaque. The peculiar color of the hen's egg is owing to the yellowish oil which pervades the whole substance. The study of the hen's egg in all its stages leaves no doubt that the cells—at least those within the egg—are formed by the swelling of the yolk particles, and their subsequent growth into larger vesicles containing a fluid, in which the elements of a perfect cell are finally matured.

Fig. 20.

Fig. 21.

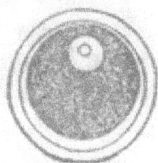

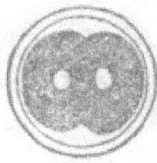

THE UNIMPREGNATED EGG after the disappearance of the germinal disk and adherent granules.

THE HUMAN EGG during segmentation into two parts.

At this stage of the ovarian egg, that is, when it has acquired the vitaline membrane, germinative vesicle and germinative dot, and has also acquired certain dimensions differing in different animals, it is, or may be, fecundated. This fecundation consists

Fig. 22.

Fig. 23.

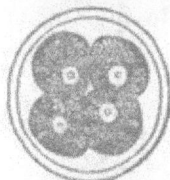

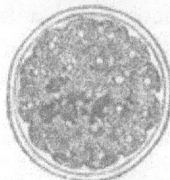

THE HUMAN EGG undergoing segmentation into four parts.

Further subdivisions of the human egg during segmentation, called the mulberry stage.

in the contact of sperm cells with the yolk bag. What the influence of that contact is, nobody has been able to trace. It is from that time that the changes date which lead toward the formation of a new being. But the egg of the hen, when fecundated, has not yet completed its growth. The hen's egg, as we know it, has a shell, and a delicate membrane lining the shell, and a layer of white albumen surrounding the yolk. All these parts are formed after the egg has been fecundated.

The egg, as we have seen, is, in its incipient condition, only an organic granule arising between the structural cells of the ovary. It grows there and acquires a remarkable complication before it has completed its successive phases as an egg. Not until it has reached the state as that of the perfect egg does it receive the contact of the spermatic cells from which dates the formation of a new being, either male or female. This in itself is a strange thing—that a mother produces, not necessarily a being like herself, but quite as often beings so unlike herself in structure, as to be endowed with all the peculiarities of the male sex.

Fig. 24.

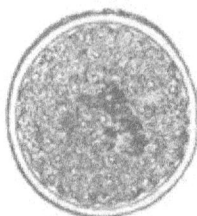

The latter stage of segmentation of the human egg.

There is one feature in the growth of the egg of which I have as yet said nothing. The yolk, that homogeneous substance which fills the vitelline membrane, in which swim the germinative vesicle and germinative dot, must undergo a very remarkable change before it can give rise to the new individual. It is self-kneading, broken by the process of its own growth into a smaller or larger number of distinct fragments. This breaking up of the whole substance which simulates disintegration ends in a recementation; these fragments reunite to form the mass out of which the new germ is to be developed. This process is known as segmentation, and has been observed in the eggs of all animals. It has been studied in mammalia, in birds, in reptiles, in

Fig. 25.

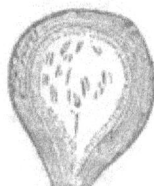

HUMAN OVUM.
A perfectly normal human ovum, twenty-one days after impregnation, inclosed in its decidua. Size of nature.

Fig. 26.

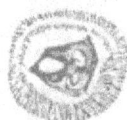

HUMAN OVUM LAID OPEN.
The ovum, with the decidua laid open; the embryo, about two lines long, closely surrounded by the amnion, is seen through the division of the chorion.

fishes, among articulates, among mollusks and radiates. This process may or may not be initiated by fecundation. There are some animals in which the first appearance of segmentation may precede fecundation; others in which it is always subsequent to fecundation ; in no animal is the process known to be completed without fecundation. Neither does it take place in all animals in the same manner.

Let us take the highly magnified yolk of a mammalian egg with the germinative dots already formed on the side. The vitelline membrane surrounding such a yolk is rather thicker than in a bird's egg, and forms a sort of transparent zone outside of the yolk. When the process of segmentation begins, the yolk shrinks slightly upon itself and no longer fills the vitelline membrane completely. Presently a slight indentation becomes visible on one side of the yolk, and another corresponding to it on the opposite side. This indentation grows deeper and deeper until it cuts the yolk through, and ends in its total division in two halves,

Fig. 27.

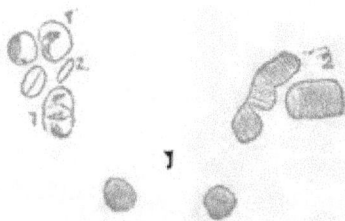

CORPUSCLET OF THE BLOOD.

The blood-corpuscles, as seen on their flat surface and edge. Congeries of blood-corpuscles in columns. In congulating, the corpuscles apply themselves to each other, so as to resemble piles of money. Below are blood globules, or cells, containing smaller cells, which are set free by the dissolution of the containing cell.

the two halves remaining, however, in close contact. While this process goes on, the germinative vesicle vanishes, if indeed it has not disappeared before. In some animals this vesicle is dissolved before the segmentation begins; in others during the process. The division of the yolk in halves being completed, the same change begins now in the two halves. Indentations are seen on either side of each half and these indentations deepen till they meet and sever the two masses of yolk ; and now, where we had one yolk mass, we have four distinct lumps side by side ; they become rounded in form, and look like four soft balls. The original yolk being thus divided in four, the same process goes on till the four are divided into eight, the eight into 16, the 16 into 32, the 32 into 64, and so on.

Beyond this it is almost impossible to track them individually; it is difficult to bring the whole yolk into the focus, so that each fragment can be counted, and if it is pressed, however slightly, the whole mass then runs together, so that no division whatever can be traced. Occasionally, however, the self-division has been followed even beyond sixty-four. By this time the yolk is transformed into a body which has much the appearance of a mulberry, and this condition of the yolk has been called the mulberry stage. When it has become so far subdivided that every separate particle, owing to its diminutive size, is difficult of microscopic observation, even under very high power, each such particle seems like a cell, and may indeed be considered as a cell. This self-division of the yolk mass ends in an accumulation of cells which differ from those of the initiative yolk, and are the basis for the

Fig. 28.

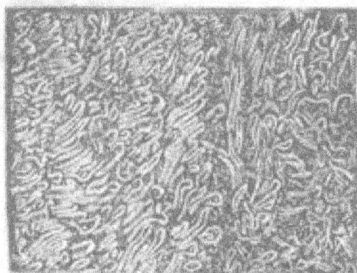

DISTRIBUTION OF CAPILLARY BLOOD-VESSELS IN SKIN OF FINGER.

formation of the new being; the material in fact out of which the new being is to be built.

When conception, or the fertilization of the germ has been accomplished, a great change takes place in the system of the female, in which arises a series of functions totally unknown in the male. The ovary is quiescent. No germs are developed and expelled during the nine months of gestation; nor, normally, during the whole period of nursing. The mammary glands become active, and, in many cases, the breasts are filled with milk at an early period of pregnancy. Life flows to the bosom instead of the ovaries. As the ovarian action is suspended, there is no occasion for the menstrual excitement and evacuation. Its cessation is therefore the earliest, and, in the healthy female, the surest sign that conception has taken place. And where there is health, and the entire absence of amative excitement, as there always should be during the whole perion of gestation and lactation—from the beginning of pregnancy until the child is weaned—the menses are suspended.

Fig. 29.

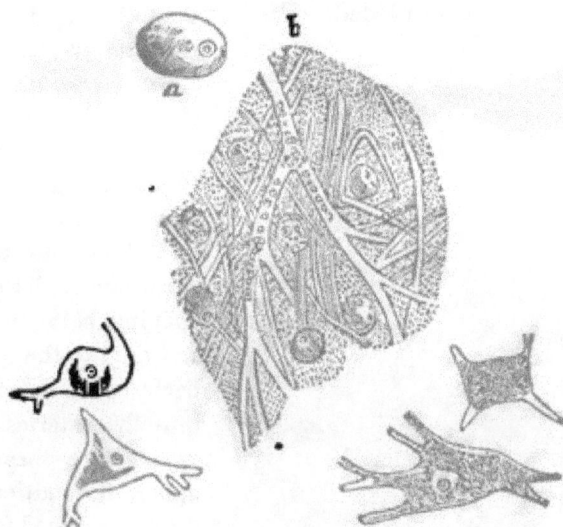

BRAIN AND NERVE.

Primitive fibres and ganglionic globules of human brain, after Purkinje. A, ganglionic globules lying among varicose nerve-tubes and blood-vessels, in substance of optic thalamus; a, globule more enlarged; b, small vascular trunk. B, B. globules with variously-formed prolongations, from dark portion of crus cerebri.

Foetal life has some remarkable peculiarities, which we may well consider. The formation of germs in the ovaries, their periodical development and expulsion, their impregnation or fecundation by spermatozoa formed in corresponding male organs; their extreme minuteness and rapid development into all the complexities of our wondrous organization, constitute a series of mysteries. But the mode of fœtal existence is strangely different from that of the infant from the moment it comes into the world. The fœtus cannot breathe. Its lungs are useless— no blood is thrown into them except what is necessary for their growth, and no air penetrates them, for the fœtus swims in a liquid. The fœtal heart has an open communication between the two auricles which is closed at birth. The blood of the infant gets its supply of oxygen from the blood of the mother by means of the placenta, or afterbirth. The lungs of the mother breathe for herself and her offspring during pregnancy, so that pure air is then more than ever needed. The blood of the child, fed and purified by that of the mother, passes from the placenta through the umbilical vein to its liver, and thence into the right auricle of the heart, and from that into the left auricle through the fœtal opening between them, and then to the left ventricle, and is expelled into the arteries which supply the head and upper extremities with the purest blood for their more rapid development.

Fig. 30.

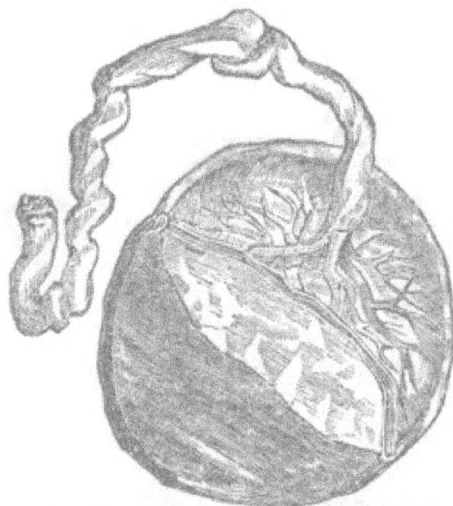

THE PLACENTA AND UMBILICAL CORD.
Showing the distribution of vessels on the
fœtal side of the placenta.

From the head and arms the blood returns into the right auricle, from which it passes to the right ventricle. In the adult it would now pass into the lungs, but in the fœtus it is carried by a special artery, afterwards obliterated, into the descending aorta, and sent partly to the lower extremities, and partly to the placenta, to be purified by contact, through thin membranes, with the blood of the mother.

Here we have a special machinery, an opening in the heart which is closed at birth, lungs solid and useless, arteries and veins most important in the fœtus, but at birth obliterated, and an organ expelled at birth after the infant, which in its fœtal life performs the function of both stomach and lungs, furnishing the matter of blood, and also the oxygen for its purification and vivification.

There is striking similarity of all forms of embryo. A fish, a reptile, a bird, a quadruped, a man are all Vertebrates by their plan of structure and by their mode of development, and yet they are entirely distinct as members of different classes of the vertebrate type. The structural plan for all Vertebrates consists of a central axis with a solid, mostly bony arch, above, inclosing the nervous system, and a similar arch below, inclosing the organs of digestion, reproduction, circulation and respiration. A glance at their embryology will show us that they are united by their development as closely as by their anatomy. Suppose we have here the egg of a vertebrate, of any vertebrate, a fish, a reptile, a bird, or a mammal; the result of the segmentation is the formation of a layer of more completely kneaded yolk substance on one side of the yolk. One end of this layer thickens more than the other. Along the middle, a slight depression is formed, not by a sinking of the centre, but in consequence of the rising and swelling of the sides which leads to the formation of a kind of furrow. It is in fact only the folding upward of the upper margins; and this goes on till the margins meet and inclose a cavity. This depression in the longitudinal axis of the germ is the beginning of the arch within-which the

Fig. 31.

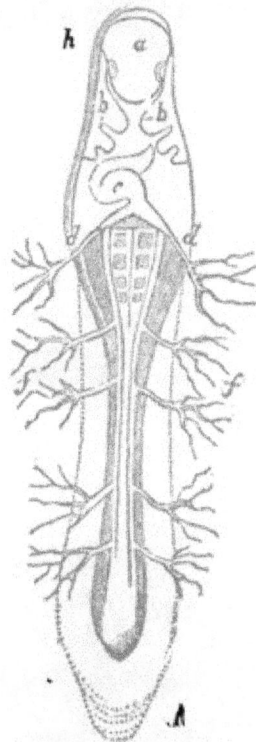

EMBRYO OF THE DOG.

This represents the same embryo as shown in the ovum of Fig. 21, highly magnified, seen from the abdominal aspect. a, is the vertex, or top, of the head. b, b, are the branchiæ, like the gills of fishes, which all mammals, man included, at one stage resemble. c, is the rudimental heart, appearing as a contorted tube. d, d, Veins of the germinal membrane. f, f, Arteries of the same, springing from the two aortas. h, h, Germinal membrane. The human embryo, at this stage, is precisely similar.

nervous system is contained. Then the lower margins of the
germ layer fold downward in the same way till they also meet and
form the lower cavity in which the other systems of organs are
inclosed. Here a little fold occurs which is the first sketching

Fig. 32.

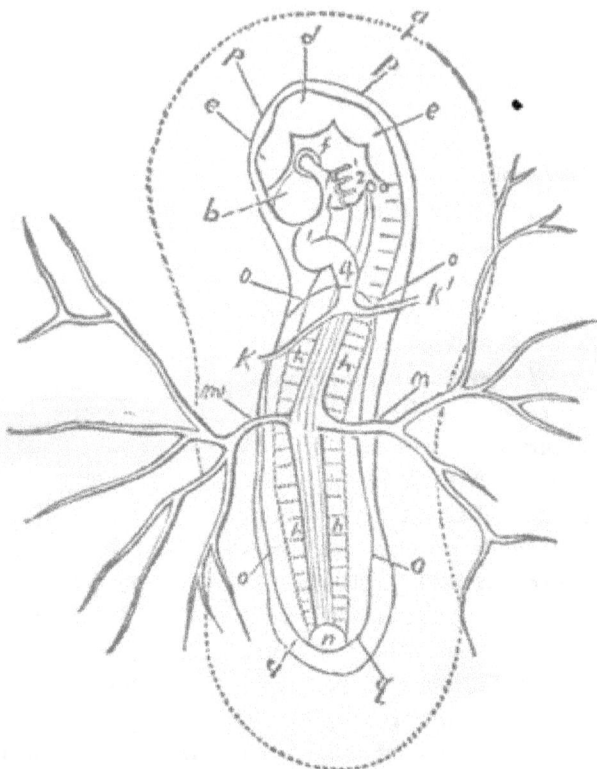

EMBRYO CHICKEN.

A magnified embryo of **the chick, four** lines long ; time, middle of the
third day. b, c, d, represent the hemispheres of the brain ; c. the cerebellum and medulla oblongata ; h, h, vertebral lamina; f, ventricle of the heart,
m, m, arteries of the blastoderma; o, o, boundaries of the abdomen ; g, opening of the ear ; f, the eye, formed first with a wide cleft. This also resembles, in all respects, the human embryo, at the same stage of development,
but at a much later period.

out of the eye ; here another fold, the first indication of the ear;
here transverse fissures are developed which are to be the gills ;
for gills exist in all vertebrates, including man, in the embryonic
state. As the development goes on, the germ rises more and more
above the yolk, the connection becomes less and less, the yolk

hangs like a bag below the body, and either is slowly or more rapidly absorbed into it, as the case may be, in different vertebrates, and the little animal is finally freed from all connection

Fig. 33.

Fig. 48 shows a further advanced embryo, with an apparatus of nutrition, called the alantois, *a*, with the umbilical vessels, *b*, branching over it. *c*. The external ear. *d*. Cerebellum. *e*. Corpora quadrigemina. *f*. Hemispheres. The eye is very large, and far advanced ; the mouth begins to take the shape of a bill, and the legs and wings are sprouting.

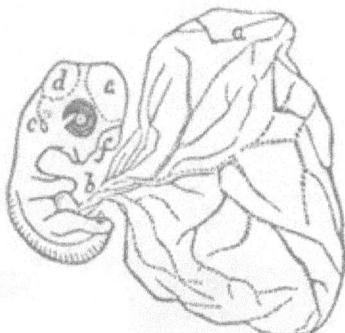

EMBRYO FOWL OF EIGHT DAYS.

with the parent. Compare a number of vertebrates from different classes in different stages of growth, and you will be astonished at their great resemblance. Take them, for instance, at an early stage of embryonic life, before the germ rises very high above the yolk. At that time blood-vessels extent over the whole yolk, some of which bring the blood to the heart, while others

Fig. 34.   Fig. 35.

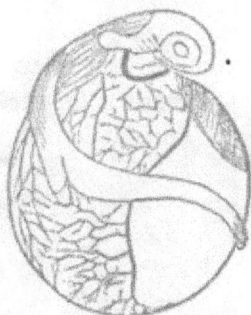

Circulation of a FISH before hatching.

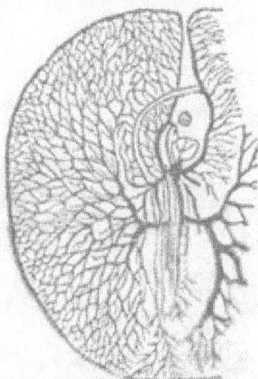

Circulation of CHICKEN at an early stage of growth in the egg.

distribute it to all parts of the surface. At this point of the development there are two great vessels from which the blood cir-

Fig. 36.

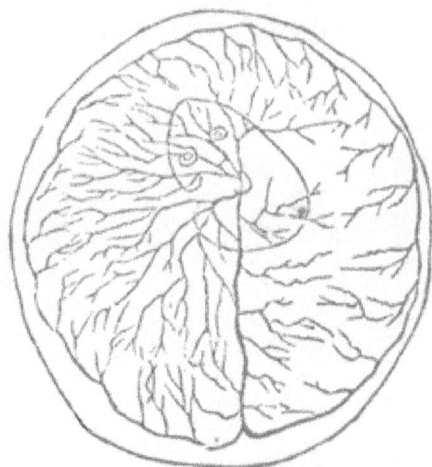

Circulation of Embryo of GUINEA PIG, on the
18th day of gestation.

Fig. 37.

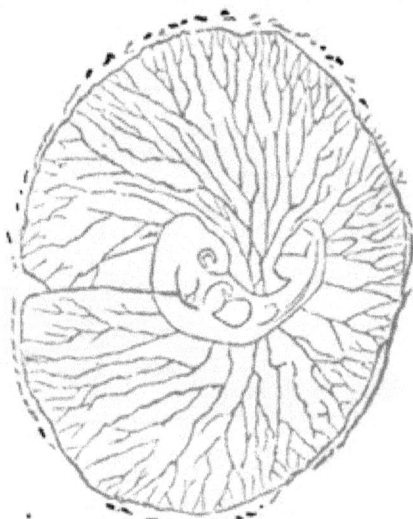

Circulation of the SNAPPING TURTLE, at an
early stage of growth in the egg.

culates symmetrically on either side of the body, while both finally unite in a circular vessel. Whether wo take a turtle, a snake, a bird, or a mammal at this phase of development, the difference in their circulation is very slight. Only very careful and detailed drawings, such as are here reproduced from the works of Rathke, Tander, Bischoff, and Agassiz, give it to you.

The body of the snake is hardly more elongated than that of the turtle; the form tapers into a tail in both, but not more in one than in the other. A young fish exhibits the same traits of physiognomy which wo observe as characteristic of the embryo of the reptiles, the birds or the mammalia. There is, in fact, no more difference between these different embryos than between the young star fish, the young jelly fish, and the young coral. The Vertebrates, like the Radiates, pass through an uninterrupted series of changes from the first formation of the germ to the completion of its growth, which are throughout parallel to one another. How, then, does it come that the germ of a turtle always produces a turtle, the germ of a snake always a snake, the germ of a dog always a dog, the germ of a man always a human being, if there be not something superior to these physical resemblances controlling all growth throughout the civilized world.

Fig. 38.

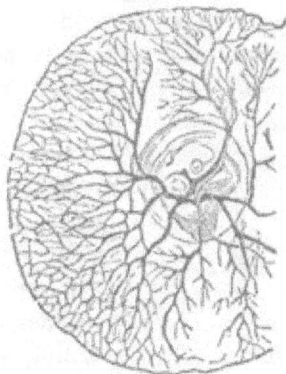

Circulation of a SNAKE, at an early stage of growth in the egg.

CHAPTER VI.

PREGNANCY.—LABOR.—PARTURITION.

Perhaps there is no more eventful period in the history of woman than that in which she first becomes conscious that the existence of another being is dependent upon her own, and that she carries about with her the first tiny rudiments of an immortal soul.

The signs of pregnancy are various. Many females are troubled with colic pains, creeping of the skin, shuddering, and fainting fits immediately on conception taking place. Where such symptoms occur immediately after connection, they are a certain indication of impregnation.

A remarkable change takes place in the face in most cases, varying in time from three days to three months. The eyes are dull and heavy, and present a glassy appearance—the nose pinched up, the skin becomes pale and livid, and the whole countenance appears as if five or ten years advance in life had been taken at a single step.

Another important and remarkable sign, and one the most to be relied on, is an increase of the size of the neck. This often occurs at a very early period, and many females, by keeping a careful daily measurement of the neck, can always tell when they are pregnant.

A suppression of the menstrual flow is another strong presumptive sign. It is true, a partial flow of the menses often occurs after pregnancy, from the lower part of the womb, but when the flow is suddenly stopped without any apparent cause, pregnancy is generally the predisposing cause.

Soon after conception, the stomach often becomes affected with what is called morning sickness. On first awaking the female feels as well as usual, but on rising from her bed qualmishness begins, and, perhaps while in the act of dressing, retching and vomiting takes place.

This symptom may occur almost immediately after conception ; but it most frequently commences for the first time between two and three weeks after. Now and then it is experienced only the last six weeks or two months of pregnancy, when it is attended generally with much distress and discomfort. It continues, more or less, during the first half of pregnancy, and subsides about the time the movements of the child begin to be felt.

Changes in the breast are generally considered as strong signs of pregnancy. When two months of pregnancy have been completed, an uneasy sensation of throbbing and stretching fullness is experienced, accompanied with tingling about the middle of the breasts, centering in the nipples. A sensible alteration in their appearance soon follows—they grow larger and more firm. The nipple becomes more prominent, and the circle around its base altered in color and structure, constituting what is called the areola ; and, as pregnancy advances, milk is secreted.

The period of gestation, at which these changes may occur, varies much in different females. Sometimes, with the exception of the secretion of the milk, they are recognized very soon after conception ; in other instances, particularly in females of a weakly and delicate constitution, they are hardly perceptible until pregnancy is far advanced, or even drawing toward its termination.

The changes in the form and size of the breast may be the result of causes unconnected with pregnancy. They may enlarge in consequence of marriage, from the individual becoming stout and fat, or from accidental suppression of the monthly flow.

The changes which take place in the nipple and around its base, are of the utmost value as an evidence of pregnancy.

About the sixth or seventh week after conception has taken place, if the nipple be examined, it will be found becoming turgid and prominent, and a circle forming around its base, of a color deeper in its shade than rose or flesh color, slightly tinged with a yellowish or brownish hue, and here and there upon its surface will be seen little prominent points from about ten to twenty in number. In the progress of the next six or seven weeks these changes are fully developed, the nipple becoming more prominent and turgid than ever, the circle around it of larger dimensions, the skin being soft, bedewed with a slight degree of moisture, frequently staining the linen in contact with it ; the little prominences of larger size, and the color of the whole very much deepened.

Calculations of the duration of pregnancy, founded upon what has been observed to occur after casual intercourse, or perhaps a single act, in individuals who can have no motive to tell us what is false, are likely to be correct. The conclusion drawn from these is, that labor usually, but not invariably, comes on about 280 days after conception, a mature child being sometimes born before the expiration of the forty weeks, and at other times not until that time had been exceeded by several days. A case is on record where the pregnancy existed 287 days. In this case, the labor did not take place until that period had elapsed from the departure of the husband for the East Indies, consequently the period might have been longer than 287 days.

Childbirth is a natural process, and however complicated and painful habits or disease have made it, yet the work must be left to Nature. Any efforts to assist or hurry matters will only end in harm. The only cases where interference is justifiable is where her powers are exhausted, or some malformation exists or malpresentation occurs. When labor is about to commence, the womb descends into the bottom of the belly, and the motions and weight of the child will be felt much lower down than usual. If in a natural position, the head will fall down to the mouth of the womb, and press upon it. This drives forward the membranes which retain the water at the orifice, and at the proper moment · they break, and labor then commences.

Labor is caused by involuntary contractions of the uterus and abdominal muscles. By their force the liquor amnii flows out, the head of the foetus is engaged in the pelvis, it goes through it, and soon passes out by the valve, the folds of which disappear. These different phenomena take place in succession, and continue a certain time; they are accompanied with pains more or less severe, with swelling and softening of the soft parts of the pelvis and external genital parts, and with an abundant mucous secretion in the cavity of the vagina. All these circumstances, each in its own way, favor the passage of the foetus.

It is proper here to remark that parturition is not necessarily either painful or dangerous. It is well known that women in an uncivilized state suffer very little pain or disablement in bringing forth children, generally neither pregnancy nor labor interrupt the ordinary avocation of the mother, except for an hour or two at the birth itself. The suffering and debilitating influences that often attend child-birth now, is caused by our unnatural modes of living, and non-attention to the laws of health. Numerous well authenticated instances are known, where women, who had previously suffered with severe labor in child-birth, have, by attention to health and diet as here indicated, been delivered of fine healthy children with comparative ease.

From the beginning of pregnancy, more than ordinary care should be used in taking regular exercise in the open air, being careful to avoid fatigue and over-exertion; during the whole period of pregnancy every kind of agitating exercise, such as running, jumping, jolting in a carriage, dancing, lifting heavy weights, and plunging in cold water, should be carefully avoided, as well as the passions being kept under perfect control.

The diet must chiefly consist of fruits and farinacious food, as sago, tapioca, rice, &c. In proportion as a woman subsists upon aliment which is free from earthy and boney matter, will she avoid pain and danger in delivery; hence the more ripe fruit, acid fruit in particular, and the less of other kinds of food, but particularly of bread or pastry of any kind, is consumed, the less will be the danger and sufferings of child-birth. Nearly all kinds of fruit possess two hundred times less ossifying principle than bread, or anything else made of wheaten flour.

Honey, molasses, sugar, butter, oil, vinegar, etc., when unadultered, are entirely free from earthy matter. Common salt, pepper, coffee, cocoa, spices, and many drugs are much worse than wheaten flour, in their harding and bone-forming tendency, and should therefore be avoided. The drink should be tea or lemonade made with water, soft and clear, and, where practicable, distilled.

No mother who has adopted this mode of living, but has blessed the knowledge of it, and it has saved many a young mother much needless terror.

CHAPTER VII.

• LOVE AND MARRIAGE.

The attraction of the sexes for each other, though based upon the dual principle of generation which pervades the living world, and which has its analogies in the attractive forces of matter, yet pervades the whole being. Love is not merely the instinctive desire of physical union, which has for its object the continuation of the species; it belongs to the mind as well as to the body; it warms, invigorates, and elevates every sentiment, every feeling, and in its highest, purest, most diffusive form, unites us to God, and all creatures in him.

All love is essentially the same, but modified according to its objects, and by the character of the one who loves. The love of children for their parents, of parents for offspring, brotherly and sisterly love, the love of friendship, of charity, and the fervor of religious love, are modifications of the same sentiment—the attraction that draws us to our kindred, our kind—that binds together all races, and humanity itself, resting on the Fatherhood of God, and the brotherhood of man. It is but natural that this love should vary in degrees. Attractions are proportional to proximity. Family is nearer than country; we prefer our own nation to the rest of the race.

FIG. 39.

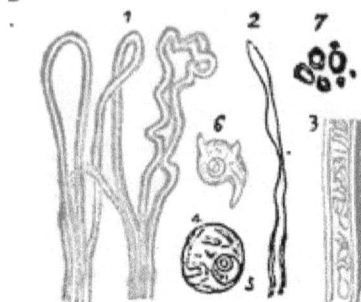

Fig. 39 represents the microscopic elements of the
nervous structure. 1. Mode of termination of white
nerve-fibers in loops; three of these loops are simple, the fourth is convoluted. The latter is found in
situations where a high degree of sensation existsf.
2. A white nerve-fiber from the brain, showing the
varicose or knotty appearance produced by traction
or pressure. 3. A white nerve-fiber enlarged to show
its structure, a tubular envelope and a contained
substance—neurilemma and neurine. 4. A nerve-
cell, showing its composition of a granular looking
capsule and granular contents. 5. Its nucleus containing a nucleolus. 6. A nerve-cell, from which
several processes are given off; it contains also a
nucleated nucleus. 7. Nerve-granules.

FIG. 40.

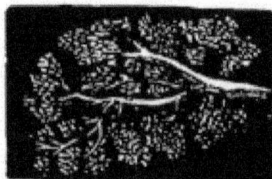

Origin of the Milk Ducts.

FIG. 41.

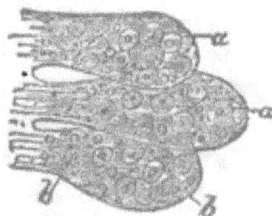

Ultimate Follicles of the
Mammary Glands.

a, a. The Secreting Cells,
b, b, the Nuclei.

Each individual has also his own special attractions and repulsions. There is love at first sight, and friendship at first sight. We feel some persons pleasant to us; to be near them is a delight. Generally such feelings are mutual—like flows to like ; or, as often, perhaps, differences fit into each other. We seek sympathy with our own tastes and habits ; or we find in others what we lack. Thus the weak rest upon the strong, the timid are fond of the courageous, the reckless seek guidance of the prudent, and so on.

The sentiment of love for the opposite sex—tender, romantic, passionate, begins very early in life. Fathers and daughters, mothers and sons, have a special fondness for each other, as also have brothers and sisters ; but the boy soon comes to admire some one, generally older than himself who is not a relation. Very little girls find a hero in some friend of an elder brother. Fondness for cousins generally comes more from opportunity than natural attraction, though a cousin may have very little appearance of family relation. The law appears to be that free choice seeks the diverse and distant. A stranger has always a better chance with the young ladies of any district than the young men with whom they have always been acquainted. Savages seek their wives out of their own tribe.

It is my belief that, naturally—I mean in a state of pure and unperverted nature, but developed, cultivated and refined by education—every man loves womanhood itself, and all women so far as they approximate to his ideal ; and that, in the same way, every woman loves manhood, and is attracted and charmed by all its gentle, noble, and heroic manifestations. By such a man, every woman he meets is reverenced as a woman, accepted as a friend, loved as a mother, sister, daughter, or it may be, cherished in a more tender relation, which should be at first, and may always remain, pure and free from any sensual desire. Such love may have many objects, each attracting the kind and degree of affection which it is able to inspire. Such love of men for women, and women for men, may be free, and will be free, just in the degree in which it is freed from the bondage of sensual passion. Such love has a direct tendency to raise men above the control of their senses. The more such love one has, and the more it is diffused, the less the liability to sink into the lower and disorderly loves of the sensual life.

The idea that every attraction, every **attachment,** every love between the sexes, must **lead** to marriage—that no love can be **tolerated but with that end in view, is a very false and** mischievous **one. It deprives men and women of** the strength and happiness **they might have in pure friendships and** pure loves, and it leads **to a multitude of false and bad marriages.** Two persons are drawn **together** by strong attractions and tender sentiments for each other, who have no **more** right **to be** married than if they were brother and sister, but who have the same right to love each other. But their true sentiments for each other, and consequent **relation to each other, are not understood** by those around them, **and perhaps not by themselves. They are** urged, by the misap- **prehension of others, by their expectation, by** ignorant gossip, • **by the prejudice of society based upon low and sensual estimates of life, to** marry ; they **find often that** they must either marry or lose the happiness they have in each other's society, and they make the irrevocable mistake.

When it is understood that there are other **loves than that** of marriage—when the special attraction **that justifies union for** life, and the begetting **of offspring, is discriminated from all** the **other attractions that may bring two souls into very near and tender relations to each other, there will be more happi-** • **ness in the world, and 'fewer incomplete, imperfect, and there-** fore more or **less unhappy marriages. Nothing can be more** detestable **than that playing with fire,** which goes by **the name** of flirtation; **but there are men and women** who have the happi- **ness of loving, and of being tenderly and devotedly loved, by persons of the opposite sex—loved** purely, nobly, **and** happily, **without injury, and with great good.** Where such loves are ac- companied by perfect **trust in the** goodness, purity, truth, and honor of the beloved, there **can be no** jealousy—no desire for sel- fish absorption—no fear of deprivation of any right. There is **no** reason why a husband or a wife should limit the range **of pure and spiritual** affections to near relatives. **The man who can love a sister or sisters are often loved, may love in the same way, or as purely, any woman who might be his sister. As men and** women **learn to purify** their lives, the world will grow more tolerant, and love will become more **universal. The tender and** fervent **exhor-** tations to mutual love, **to be found in the** Gospels and Epistles of the New Testament, are now almost without a meaning. But they had a meaning to those to whom they were addressed, and when we are better Christians, and bring our lives to the purity of Christian morality, they will have a meaning to us, and we shall learn that in a sense we have not dreamed of, God is Love.

In the human race all circumstances point to monogamy as the law, or natural condition. Males and females are born in almost exactly equal numbers. If there are two or three per cent. more of males than females, the risks of life with males soon make the number even. Therefore, as a rule, no man can have more than one wife without robbing his neighbor. Polygamy is therefore a manifest injustice, and may become the most grievous of all monopolies.

Children are the most helpless of all young creatures, and require the care of parents for the longest period. The care of a husband for his wife, and of a father for his child, is an evident necessity. The proper care and education of a single child should extend over at least fifteen years, and that of a family may reach to thirty years, or throughout the greater part of an ordinary life. During all periods of pregnancy, child-bearing, nursing, and the education and care of a family, every woman has a right to the sympathy, sustaining love, and constant aid of her husband. No man has the right to desert or leave helpless, or even dependent upon others, except in extraordinary cases, the mother of his children.

Marriage, like celibacy, should be a matter of vocation. The special object of marriage is to have children—the co-operating motive is that two persons, drawn to each other by a mutual affection, may live helpfully and happily together. A selfish marriage for its merely animal gratifications—a marriage in which strength, health, usefulness, often life itself, are sacrificed to sensuality and lust—is a desecration of a holy institution, and somewhat worse in its consequences than promiscuous profligacy, for the consequences of that may not fall upon one's children and posterity.

There are many persons who have no right to marry. There should be a kind and amount of love that will justify and sanctify such a relation. There should be a pure motive, and a fixed intention of making the relation what it ought to be to husband, wife, and children. There should be a reasonable assurance of the power to provide for a family. There should be that amount of health—that freedom from bodily and mental disease—that physical and moral constitution which will give a reasonable prospect of children whose lives will be a blessing to themselves and to society.

Where there is deformity of body or an unhappy peculiarity of mind or temper liable to be inherited, people should not marry, or if they live together, should resign the uses of marriage. People should conscientiously refrain from propagating hereditary diseases. Persons near of kin are wisely forbidden to marry, for there is in such cases the liability of imperfect generation—the production of blind, deaf, idiotic or insane offspring.

Should marriage be for life? As a rule, undoubtedly. Every real, proper, true marriage must be. It takes a lifetime for a husband and wife to make a home, and rear, and educate, and provide for a family of children. But how if people make mistakes and find that they are not suitably married? These are mistakes very difficult to remedy. If a man, after deliberately making his choice of a woman, ceases to love her, how can he honorably withdraw from his relation to her, and enter upon another, when she still loves him, and is ready to fulfil her part of the contract? Laws cannot very well provide for mistakes. If the distaste for each other be mutual, and both parties desire to separate, a separation may of course be permitted, but it is a serious question whether two such persons can go into the world and find new partners, with justice to the rest. The law which permits of no divorce certainly bears hard upon individual cases, but if it leads to greater seriousness and care in forming such relations, it may be, on the whole, the best thing for society that it should be strictly observed.

CHAPTER VIII.

WHEN TO MARRY. — HOW TO SELECT A PARTNER ON RIGHT
PRINCIPLES.

The proper age to marry is a somewhat vexed question, but
needlessly so, because that age varies much, according to temper-
ment and other circumstances relating to the individual. Although,
after puberty, the sexual organs are capable of reproduction, yet
it by no means follows that they should be used for that purpose.
Their early activity is intended for the perfection of the body and
mind, and not for the continuation of the species. Very early
marriages, therefore, should be avoided, because the nervous force
expended in amative indulgence is imperatively required in both
sexes, for developing the physical and mental faculties. The zoospermes produced by the male in the first years of puberty are
inferior in power, and less capable of producing healthy offspring
than those of maturer years. The early germs, also, of the female
are less fitted for fecundation than those that appear latter in life.
Nature evidently intending these early efforts to be used on the
individuals themselves, in building up their bodies, strengthening
their minds, and preparing them to reproduce their species in
maturer years. There is a serious day of reckoning for early indulgence; for precocious persons—unless their constitutions are
as powerful as their desires—who give way to their passions at
their first exactions, barter their youth for their enjoyment, and
are old and weary of the world at an age when people of more
moderate habits are only in the meridian of pleasure and existence.

Generally, the best age to marry, where the health is perfect,
is from twenty-one to twenty-five in the male, and from eighteen
to twenty-one in the female. As a general rule, marriages earlier
than this are injurious and detrimental to health. Men who
marry too young, unless they are of cold and phlegmatic constitutions, and thus moderate in their conduct, become partially
bald, dim of sight, and lose all elasticity of limb, in a few years;
while women, in a like position, rarely have any bloom on their
cheek or fire in their eye, by the time they are twenty-five. And

all profound physiologists agree that, from the same cause, the mental faculties suffer in the same ratio.

A medium, however, is to be observed. It is not well to differ till middle age the period of connubial intercourse ; for too tedious spinstership is as much calculated to hasten the decay of beauty, as too early a marriage. Hence, there is rarely any freshness to be seen in a maiden of thirty ; while the matron of that age, if her life has been a happy one, and her hymenial condition of not more than ten years' standing, is scarcely in the hey-day of her charms. And the same rule will apply with equal force to the other sex ; for, after the first prime of life, bachelors decay and grow old much faster than married men.

The rich are qualified for marriage before the poor. This is owing to the superiority of their aliment ; for very nutritious food, and the constant use of wines, coffee, etc., greatly assists in developing the organs of reproduction ; whereas the food generally made use of among the peasantry of most countries—as vegetables, corn, milk, etc.—retards their growth. Owing to this difference of diet, the daughter of a man of wealth, who keeps a good table, will be as adequate to certain duties of married life at eighteen, as the daughter of a humble peasant at twenty-one. Singular as it may seem, it is none the less true, that love-novels, amorous conversations, playing parlor games for kisses, voluptuous pictures, waltzing, and, in fact, all things having a tendency to create desire, assist in promoting puberty, and preparing young persons for early marriage. Those who reach this estate, however, by artificial means, and much before the natural period, will have to suffer for it in after-life.

The female who marries before the completion of her womanhood—that is, before her puberty is established—will cease to grow, and probably become pale and delicate ; the more especially if she becomes pregnant soon after marriage. A person who is thus circumstanced, will also be liable to abortions, and painful deliveries. Marriage, unless under very peculiar circumstances, should not take place until two or three years after the age of puberty. Many instances could be cited of the injurious effects resulting from not observing this rule. The case of the son of Napoleon I. is a notable instance, who, at the age of fifteen or sixteen, began his career of sexual indulgence, which ended his life at the early age of twenty-one years. He was an amiable, inoffensive, and studious youth—beloved by his grandfather and the whole Austrian Court ; and though the son of the most energetic man that modern times has produced, yet, from his effeminate life, he scarcely attracted the least public attention.

Let me, therefore, advise the male reader to keep his desires in leading strings until he is at least twenty-one, and the female not to enter within the pale of wedlock until she is past her eighteenth year ; but after those periods marriage is their proper sphere of action, and one in which they must play a part, or suffer actual pain, as well as the loss of one of the greatest of earthly pleasures.

Marriages are most happy, and most productive of handsome and healthy offspring, when the husband and wife differ, not only in mental conformation, but in bodily construction. A melancholy man should mate himself with a sprightly woman, and vice versa ; for otherwise they will soon grow weary of the monotony of each other's company. By the same rule should the choleric and the patient be united, and the ambitious and the humble ; for the opposites of their natures not only produce pleasurable excitement, but each keeps the other in a wholesome check. In the size and form of the parties, the same principles hold good. Tall women are not the ideals of beauty to tall men ; and if they marry such, they will soon begin to imagine greater perfections in other forms than in those of their own wives. And this is well ordered by Nature, to prevent the disagreeable results which are almost certain to grow out of unions where the parties have a strong resemblance.

For instance : tall parents will probably have children taller than either, and mental imbecility is the usual attendant of extreme size. The union of persons prone to corpulency, of dwarfs, ¶ etc., would have parallel results ; and so, likewise, of weakly or attenuated couples. The tall should marry the short—the corpulent the lean—the choleric the gentle—and so on ; and the tendency to extremes in the parents will be corrected in the offspring.

Apart from these considerations, there are reasons why persons of the same disposition should not be united in wedlock. An amiable wife to a choleric man, is like oil to troubled waters ; an ill-tempered one will make his life a misery and his home a hell, The man of studious habits should marry a woman of sense and spirit rather than of erudition, or the union will increase the monotony of his existence, which it would be well for his health and spirits to correct by a little conjugal excitement; and the man of gloomy temperament will find the greatest relief from the dark forebodings of his mind in the society of a gentle, but lively and smiling partner.

However, in some particulars the dispositions and constructions of married people must assimilate, or they will have but few enjoyments in common. The man of full habits and warm nature had better remain single than unite his destinies with a woman whose heart repulses the soft advancements of love; and the sanguine female, in whose soul love is the dominant principle, should avoid marriage with a very phlegmatic person, or her caresses, instead of being returned in kind, will rather excite feelings of disgust. Thus the discriminations to be made in the choice of a partner are extremely nice.

Nature generally assists Art in the choice of partners. We instinctively seek in the object of our desires the qualities which we do not possess ourselves. This is a most admirable arrangement of Providence, as it establishes an equilibrium, and prevents people from tending to extremes; for it is known that unions of dwarfs are fruitful of dwarfs; that giants proceed from the embrace of giants; and that the offspring of parents alike irritable, alike passive, alike bashful, etc., inherit the prominent qualities of both to such a degree as to seriously interfere with their prospects in the world.

It has another advantage. Through its means "every eye forms its own beauty;" hence, what one person rejects is the beau ideal of another's conceptions; and thus we are all provided for.

In fine, with man as with animals, the best way to improve the breed is to cross it—for the intermarriage of like with like, and relative with relative, not only causes man to degenerate, but, if the system became universal, would in time bring the human race to a termination altogether.

A male or female with a very low forehead should carefully avoid marriage with a person of like conformation, or their offspring will, in all probability, be weak-minded, or victims to partial idiocy.

The system of **crossing is so perfect,** that marriages between persons, natives of different countries, are likely to be **pleasant** and fruitful. Speaking on this subject an English writer says : "The Persians have been so improved by introducing foreigners to breed from, that they have completely succeeded in washing out the stain of **their** Mongolian origin." **And the same** author adds to the effect, that in those parts **of Persia where there** is no foreign intercourse, the inhabitants are sickly and stunted ; **while** in those that **are** frequented **by strangers, they are large and** healthy.

To **make what is called a "handsome couple,"** the female should be about three inches less than the male ; and **the parties** should be proportionably developed throughout their system.

"A well-formed woman," says a modern physiologist, "should have her head, shoulders, and chest small and compact ; arms **and** limbs relatively **short ;** her haunches apart ; her hips elevated ; **her abdomen large, and her thighs** voluminous. Hence, she should taper from **the centre up and down. Whereas, in a** well-formed man the shoulders are more **prominent than the hips.** Great hollowness of the back, the pressing **of the thighs against** each **other** in walking, **and** the elevation **of one hip above the** other, are indications of the malformations of **the pelvis."**

From the same writer I take the following, which is applicable here. It is very correct in its estimates of beauty in both sexes : "The length of the neck should be proportionably less in the male than in the female, because the dependance of the mental system on **the vital one** is naturally connected with the shorter courses of the vessels **of the neck.**

The neck should form a gradual transition between the body and head—its fullness concealing all prominences of the throat.

The shoulders should slope from **the lower part of the neck, because the reverse shows that the upper part of the chest owes its width to the bones and muscles of the shoulders.**

The upper part of the chest should be relatively short and wide, independent of the size of the shoulders, for this shows the vital organs which it contains are sufficiently developed

The waist should taper little farther than the middle of the **trunk,** and be marked, especially in the back and loins, by the **approximation of the hips.**

The waist should be narrower than the upper part of the trunk and its muscles, because the reverse indicates the expansion of the stomach, liver, and great intestines, resulting from their excessive use.

The back of woman should be more hollow than that of man; for otherwise the pelvis is not of sufficient depth for parturition.

Woman should have loins more extended than man, at the expense of the superior and inferior parts, for this conformation is essential to gestation.

The abdomen should be larger in woman than in man, for the same reason.

Over all these parts the cellular tissue, and the plumpness connected with it, should obliterate all distinct projection of muscles.

The surface of the whole female form should be characterized by its softness, elasticity, smoothness, delicacy, and polish, and by the gradual and easy transition between the parts.

The moderate plumpness already described should bestow on the organs of the woman great suppleness.

Plumpness is essential to beauty, especially in mothers, because in them the abdomen necessarily expands, and would afterwards collapse and become wrinkled.

An excess of plumpness, however, is to be guarded against. Young women who are very fat are cold, and prone to barrenness.

In no case should plumpness be so predominant as to destroy the distinctness of parts.

A male and female formed on the above models would be well matched and have fine children."

CHAPTER IX.

A SPECIAL CHAPTER TO YOUNG MEN, UPON A SPECIAL SUBJECT.

I desire young men, to enlist your earnest attention in what I now say, upon its proper consideration, will determine in a great measure, the character of your future career.

You have now arrived at that age, when you have in a large degree to act on your own responsibility, and take your place as a worker in the world's progress. Your childhood being passed away, your parents, friends and society now look upon you and expect you to assume your alloted portion of work as a means of securing a livelihood. No one who has health has any right to existence without doing work of some kind. To help you to fill your sphere happily, successfully and worthily, has been my object in writing this chapter. No young man who has evinced a desire for the companionship of prostitutes has ever succeeded in the end, no matter what advantages he may have had in the way of friends, fortune or talents.

I take it for granted you profess Christianity, and believe in a heaven and a hell, or a future state of rewards and punishments, according to the deeds done in the body.

To the atheist or the professional profligate, who acknowledges no law, human or divine, I do not address myself. I leave him in the hands of the living God, who will surely call him to account when he least expects it.

You find yourself in the enjoyment of life, health and strength, inhabiting a beautiful world, and surrounded by abundant means of delight and happiness; and you know, not only that you did not give yourself this life, but that you are utterly powerless to prolong it even for an instant; in fact, that you are momentarily dependant for life and all its blessings on its Divine Giver. This consideration need not in the least prevent you from the unrestrained pursuit of any innocent pleasures ; but it should lead you to be most careful to abstain from any of an opposite character.

When a mere boy you preferred the companionship of boys, and probably scorned or were ashamed to play with girls. Now on the contrary, you feel yourself powerfully attracted towards young women; and find yourself much happier in their company than in that of young men. Whence, think you, comes this remarkable change? Is it not from Him who is the only Source of life and love, and who, in His wisdom and mercy, has made the two sexes, and made them for each other? And what could be His motive in this but the desire to promote the eternal happiness of His creatures? It is, too, by this wise and beneficient provision that He secures the perpetuation of the human race in this world, and a continual addition to the host of good men made perfect in His happy kingdom above.

This new feeling you may take as a notice from God that the time is approaching when it will behoove you to look about for a maiden whom you can love with a pure affection, and whom you believe you can make happy as your wife. Attend to the voice of God thus addressed to you; or, *take the consequences.*

God, as we see, has not made us angels at once, but has placed us in this world of probation, where, associated with our fellows of various and conflicting dispositions and interests, we may form our character, and be gradually prepared for our eternal home. To assist us in this preparation, and to guide us in our course of action, we often need the counsels of a judicious and kind friend; and in this case one of our own sex may be, and often is, highly valuable. But at times there are peculiar circumstances when one of the other sex—a better half, to whom we can without reserve, unbosom ourselves—is beyond all comparison preferable. To each sex God has given qualities suited to meet the wants, as well as to enhance the joys, of the other.

Every right-minded young man, on attaining a suitable age, desires to become a husband and a father; and the prospect cheers him in his toil, and nerves his arm to greater and more persistent labor than he would be willing to undertake for himself alone. He is looking forward to provide for others far dearer to him than himself.

Now, as God knows all things, He knows what pairs are fitted for each other; indeed, we cannot doubt that He provides them..

But the world is in a fallen state—I think **you will** cordially **agree** with me here—and consequently it is often difficult, or **almost** impossible, for any of us to know who are the right parties to come together.

Suppose, however, **by some** extraordinary **means,** you should **happen to know what maiden** would become **your** wife, what would be **your thoughts and feelings if** *without marriage,* she were previously, **for a time however short, to live with another man ? Would you not think her defiled and unworthy of you ? Do not most men take the same view ? How then, think you can any** accountable being **be willing to defile a woman that is to be the wife of** another?

If you are right-minded you will, in the first place, seek **for** purity **in** your bride ; and if you are honest, and worthy of a wife, **you will take** especial care not to be her inferior in that **respect.**

The Almighty **Creator, in His love and mercy towards His** creatures, permits them **to co-operate with Him in continuing** His creation ; and hence **flow all the endearing affections and** relationships **of** home and family.

The lawful love of man for woman, and **of woman for man, is the** best and holiest affection **of** which our **nature is** susceptible; **it is** also the strongest and the most enduring, and, **as** it proceeds from God Himself, nothing can be more certain than **that the** orderly compliance with its dictates secures health and happiness here and hereafter; while, **on** the other hand, the abuse of this love as certainly entails **the loss of all** self-respect, and, unless **repented of,** eternal woe.

A man that **has been** guilty of fornication **may** afterwards **desire to contract marriage,** and **with that view may pay his** addresses **to a respectable, modest young woman ; but can he—** knowing, **as he must, his own character –do** so without a feeling of inferiority, **shame, and remorse ?** Assuming that he has seen and repented of his **wicked folly, he ought,** before taking such a **step, to** perform a mental quarantine, say of not less than **six** months; in other words, he ought for a considerable time, **to** abstain not only from lascivious acts and practices, but also from encouraging unchaste thoughts, so as to have a well-grounded assurance that he has effectually abandoned his vicious practices, and is determined for the future to pursue a virtuous course, such as may become a Christian husband and father.

Supposing you have a sister whom you tenderly love, and some man—perhaps a friend of yours—should by taking advantage of her unsuspecting credulity, succeed in seducing her, you would doubtless consider him an unprincipled villain, and deserving of the most condign punishment. If too, as is often the case, she should in consequence, although unmarried, become a mother, you know the disgrace into which she would fall, especially in the eyes of her own sex. Parents, in such cases, not unfrequently turn their backs on the child they had tenderly reared, and from whose honorable marriage they had expected a large addition to their own happiness. But suppose the victim, instead of being your sister, were only an acquaintance, or even a stranger, would not your detestation of the villany be quite as real, though perhaps not so intense?

In all such cases—and alas! they are far too numerous—the evil is one of the greatest that can befall a human being; and, although the men commonly go scatheless in the eyes of the world, are they not in the eyes of God—who alone judges rightly—as truly and lamentably fallen as the women?

In the three commandments, forbidding murder, adultery, and theft, I remark that adultery is placed between the other two; and from this I infer that the crime of an adulterer lies somewhere between that of a murderer and a thief. For does not adultery—to which fornication is the natural stepping-stone—partake of the nature of both murder and theft? To deprive a woman of her chastity is robbery of the basest description; and adultery injures or destroys the soul as certainly as poison does the body. To me it appears that the phrase, a Christian murderer, a Christian adulterer, a Christian thief, or a Christian drunkard, is a contradiction in terms; and that so long as such a character attaches to any one he is unchristianized, self-excommunicated, and utterly disqualified for heaven.

Let me here, however, add that I firmly believe there is such a thing as genuine repentance; and therefore that any one who has committed a crime, however heinous, may repent, and so become fitted for admission to the pure society in heaven. But I know full well that real repentance is both difficult and rare ; and therefore how extremely dangerous it is for any one to enter on a vicious course.

It is often easy enough to evade man's laws ; indeed, not a few of them are more honored in the breach than in the observance. Being in their very nature imperfect, they are liable to and admit of alteration and improvement. God's laws, however, are the reverse of all this. They are perfect and unalterable in their nature, are all intended and calculated to promote our good, are certain in their effects, and eternal in their operation, like Him who gave them ; and, happily, there is no escape from them. This important fact is forgotten or neglected whenever we knowingly give way to any vicious propensity. *As we sow we are certain to reap.*

In my view, it is according to God's law that a man should attach himself to one woman in that most intimate relation, Marriage, and one woman to one man, ever being careful not to do anything that would divert the affections of any one from their proper object ; for to each one God has given a right to one, and only one. It is our duty jealously to guard our own right ; and, if our practice conform to our Christian profession, we shall be as careful, to the utmost of our power, not to infringe the rights of others, especially on this most tender point. Whoever, then, commits fornication or adultery, trespasses on the domain of another, and so offends God's law, and must inevitably take the consequences ; and, recollect, the punishment that naturally follows any wicked act is ever in exact proportion to its atrocity.

Whatever some may think or say, do not you give heed to the notion that 'A reformed rake makes the best husband.' Many a youth may have fancied that he might, with little or no danger, have just a taste of intoxicating liquor, or of fornication, and give it up after a time ; forgetting that practice makes perfect— as well in a bad cause as a good one—and that a habit once acquired is very rarely got rid of : witness the number of confirmed drunkards, and permanently diseased and decayed libertines, sunk to the lowest depths of degradation. How is it, I wonder, that wo do not hear it said A reformed harlot makes the best wife'? Reform is surely as possible for women as for men. I hope and believe that many harlots do repent and reform ; but I fear a very great many more do not: for it is well known that those who have once fallen into a vicious practice, whatever it may be, are far more in danger of repeating it than those who have never entered upon it.

I am well aware that young men are liable to be tempted to stray from the path of duty in a great variety of ways, some of them most insidious and dangerous. Many have large sums of money passing through their hands, or large stocks of valuable goods, some of which they might easily take with but little chance of detection ; yet they safely pass through the trying ordeal. Sometimes they will be invited by their youthful acquaintance, of either sex, to partake of pleasures which their conscience tells them are anything but innocent. In all such cases, let them as zealously guard their own chastity as they habitually do their employer's property; and they will at the same time promote their own welfare, and do something towards bettering the condition of the world.

A casual visitor to our casinos, music-halls, and other places where loose girls and fast young men do congregate, might fancy there was no harm going on—that all was innocent amusement; but, could he follow a portion of the company when the closing time arrives, he would have great reason to change his opinion. Some of the less cautious, having drunk too freely, soon find their way to the cells of the police station ; but the greater number indulge their lustful propensities in dens of infamy where they are pretty safe from interference.

Indulgence in fornication inevitably entails no little expense— often much more than would support a family in comfort and respectability; and whence, think you, are the funds supplied ? Doubtless from some channel that should have a different and a better destination; and, when ordinary sources fail, an employer's till or cash-box, or his cheque-book is not unfrequently resorted to. Detection may not immediately follow, and the downward course is pursued till, from the magnitude of the robbery, or perhaps some trifling circumstance, it can no longer be concealed, and, at one blow, a felon's fate puts an end to the dissipation and forever blasts the prospects of the infatuated youth.

Like other vices, fornication is progressive in its nature, and has the most lamentable consequences. As petty theft is a stepping stone to burglary, and indulgence in drink to habitual drunkenness and delirium tremens, so fornication, when once entered on, may lead to adultery, and that may provoke homicide which, under the circumstances, would be deemed justifiable, as a jury would assert by their verdict; or it may lead to divorce, and bring disgrace and wretchedness to a number of innocent people and children.

One of the saddest results of fornication is the immense number of illegitimate children that are brought into the world, and who have not that parental care which they so much need, and to which they are so justly entitled.

How often young women are charged with the murder of their infants; and, although it is almost certain they are guilty of that crime, they are convicted only of concealing the birth. Who can tell the mental anguish they must have endured ere they could make up their minds to destroy their babes? In truth, it is quite enough to bring on temporary insanity, and so to justify the merciful verdict. Very probably, too, several of the jury felt self-convicted of having participated in a similar, though undiscovered, crime. In these cases, who will say that the fathers of those little innocents are less guilty than the wretched and disgraced mothers?

All vices carry their punishment with them, and this, too, with unerring certainty, although it does not always follow them swiftly. To this, which is one of God's laws, fornication is no exception. A young man may, perchance, practice it for some time with apparent impunity; or he may, on the other hand— unhappily, as he will doubtless will consider it—at once contract a disease so loathsome that he dares not avow it, but strives to conceal it; and so virluent, that it may either carry him to an early grave, or, after the doctors have done their best for him, leave him debilitated for life, a burden to himself and others. Unlike other diseases, this is deemed unfit to be spoken of in decent society; indeed, it is never alluded to, and is therefore more likely to be neglected till it has so thoroughly got hold of the system that recovery is hopeless. The sinning women, too, are equally subject to this horrible curse. *Whole wards in our hospitals and lunatic asylums are filled with its victims.* Such, however, is but the natural punishment which a merciful God permits to follow a violation or abuse of one of His most beneficient laws ; by this means plainly showing us the grievous nature of the crime. If the terrible character, and the inevitable certainty of this natural consequence of the act were known in time, it ought to be sufficient to deter any young person from vicious courses. Forewarned they would be forearmed.

In order to be convinced of the direful evils resulting from this vice, we need only look at the swarms of prostitutes that infest all our large centres of population; and, truth to tell, in proportion to their size, our villages and quiet hamlets are no less immoral. Most of these unfortunates, and their male associates too, pass much of their time in riotous enjoyment, which they mistakenly fancy to be happiness; but can any mistake be more complete, or more fatal in its consequences? They are placed in this world, endowed with faculties which will enable them to promote the well-being of those about them, and by that means at the same time to promote their own; instead of which they neglect the opportunities God affords them for the right and beneficial employment of their talents, and insanely pervert them to the destruction of their health, their wealth, and their prospects, both in this world and the next. Who that has human feelings can look at this state of things, and not be led to ask himself, 'How are the people that live in this way ever to get to heaven?' or, might we not rather say, '*How are they to be kept out of hell?*' and, recollect, even the vilest of these were once innocent children ! Moreover, however humiliating it may be to admit the fact, as surely as God is our common Father, so surely are they our brethren and sisters? Can, then, anything be more self-evident than that it is both the interest and the duty of every one of us to do all in our power to *prevent* the young from swerving from the path of virtue?

The evil effects of this vicious and debasing practice do not obtrude themselves so much on public notice in the case of men as of women; but, without staying to inquire which of the two are the greatest sufferers, it is notorious that it is a dreadful scourge in both the army and navy, many thousands of men always being in the hospital from the ravages it makes among them, a large portion of whom never are able to return to their duty: so large, indeed, is the number of victims as greatly to diminish the efficiency of our forces, and at the same time to inflict a heavy and wasteful expenditure on the country. This state of things, be it observed, implies a corresponding number of abandoned and infected women.

When a young man, instead of retiring at a proper time to his own chamber, spends his evening in revelry, and then shares the bed of a harlot, although he may manage to be at his post in the morning, and his daily associates be none the wiser, he knows that he has been guilty of conduct which is truly disgraceful, and of which he will be heartily ashamed—that is, provided he has not lost all sense of right and wrong. He has, in fact, degraded himself to the level of his paramour, for whom, too, he cannot have an atom of respect; and without respect there cannot be any love that is worthy of the name.

But, besides the injury the fornicator does to himself, that which he inflicts on the woman is not to be overlooked or forgotten. If she were a maiden whom he seduced, the injury is little, if any, less than that of taking her life. If she had previously fallen, he helps to confirm her in her vicious course, and renders her reformation and consequent return to respectable society, and also her ultimate salvation, much more difficult and far less probable.

And, if he look to his own case, what is it? The longer he follows a vicious course, the more it becomes a confirmed habit; and it would be as reasonable to expect that half a life spent in the study of languages only should qualify a man for a surgeon or an engineer, as that a life of unchastity should qualify him for heaven, into which nothing impure can enter.

It is a well-established fact, which cannot be too generally known, that parents transmit to their children propensities to good or evil, especially the latter; and they in their turn transmit them to their posterity. It is, then, highly probable, and often happens, that when parents have indulged in certain vicious practices, whatever they may be, their children will be strongly inclined to the same. The children, for instance, of a drunkard, a miser, a tyrant, &c., will be very likely to resemble their parents; and this holds true no less with a sensualist. Moreover, physical diseases, especially that which has been alluded to, are often transmitted to innocent offspring, even after the parents have believed themselves thoroughly cured. Many may, in this way, trace the origin of their diseases as well as of their vices to their ancestors.

These considerations cannot be too strongly impressed on the attention of the young who are beginning life. It is only of healthy parents that healthy children are born. If young people had a right estimate of the responsibility they were about to undertake when they marry, they would shrink with horror from the danger of contamination, and of permanent injury to their health, should they yield to unchaste practices. No action of our lives but carries with it important—ay, eternal—consequences; and therefore the evil effects resulting from fornication may be felt by generations yet unborn.

Many will, perhaps, say that fornication always existed and always will. I demur to both propositions, and maintain, on the contrary, that it did not exist at the beginning; for then God saw that all was good: and if God gives to one man the power to reform, repent, and be regenerated—which no one will deny—He will doubtless give it to any one and to all who ask for it; for He is love, and He loves every one of His creatures infinitely. We may, therefore, confidently look forward to the gradual decrease and ultimate extinction of this grievous curse of our race.

If you, my young friend, have already fallen into this sin, rely upon it you may shake it off entirely, provided you are sufficiently courageous, and look for strength to the only Fountain of all strength. As there is joy in heaven over one sinner that repenteth, so there is every encouragement for us to fight the good fight; for, although those who are against us are many and powerful, those who are on our side are both more numerous and more powerful.

Many well-intentioned people would like to keep the young ignorant of these sad and repulsive matters; so would I, if it were possible: but it is not; and I will not, therefore, pretend that I think you ignorant. Ignorance, be it remembered, is neither innocence nor security; and, on the other hand, knowledge does not involve either danger or guilt, but quite the contrary. I would then much rather help you to see this rampant vice in all its hideous deformity than attempt to conceal it from your notice.

'A little learning,' it has been well said, 'is a dangerous thing;' and, in like manner, a little knowledge respecting the relation between the sexes—especially when that knowledge has been acquired in a disorderly way—will be found to be highly dangerous; since the more valuable anything is, it is, on that very account, the more liable to be greatly abused: and it is not too much to say, that the evils and miseries resulting from the inordinate love of money or of wine—howsoever enormous and deplorable they may be—bear no comparison to those inflicted on humanity by the abuse of that intense love for the other sex which God has implanted in every human breast for the wisest, the most beneficent, and the holiest of purposes. It seems to me then to be one of the most important duties of parents to give their children clear and definite notions on these matters much earlier than is usual. Too often the young get their minds poisoned with unchaste ideas, by ignorant or ill-disposed servants, schoolfellows, and others, long before the parents think the time has arrived when it will be prudent to initiate them into such subjects.

Rely upon it fornication, in its natural consequences, is intimately connected with misery and hell, to which, indeed, it directly leads ; while, on the contrary, marriage as naturally and directly tends to happiness and heaven. Hence it behoves those parents who would wish to prevent their children from practising this sin to do their utmost to put them into a position, as early as may be, to enter upon matrimony. If they do not, and their children fall into temptation, a heavy responsibility lies at their door. By waiting, in the hope of securing the *respectability* so much sought after, there is great danger of their falling into ' *deadly* SIN.'

Perhaps you will say, ' Marriage is all very well for those who can marry, but you cannot.' I ask, Why not ? 'Because, in truth, you cannot afford it; at least your friends say so.' Now, although I have a strong objection to young persons marrying before either their minds or their bodies are fully developed, still I do advocate **early marriages; and I feel** certain that not one tenth part so **much mischief arises from them** as from entering **on a course of harlotry from which, alas! too many never emerge.**

Dr. James Hodson makes the following strong and pertinent remarks:—"Nothing can possibly prove **so** certain a preservative [from vicious habits, and the **consequent** diseases] as *early* and honorable MARRIAGE, **formed upon a real and sincere affection.** The arguments of *prudence* and *youth*, generally made use of against early marriages, are fallacious delusions, invented by the grand enemy of mankind: for Nature, both within and without, tells them they are *not* too young; and all the miseries that ever occurred from an early and proper marriage are not in comparison to the *ten-thousandth* part of those evils which a vicious course of life, **from fourteen** to twenty-one, entails upon mankind! In the *one* instance, a few difficulties in life only are the **greatest** consequence, which love and mutual affection generally overcome; but in the *other*.... It is the command of Heaven to marry, increase, and multiply: it is the **suggestion of hell to** forbid marriage, and to stir up unnatural affections in **young** people."

Burns—who well *knew* what was right— in his "Epistle to a **Young Friend,"** says:

> The sacred lowe of weel-placed love,
>   **Luxuriantly** indulge it;
> But never tempt th' *illicit rove*,
>   Tho' naething should **divulge it.**
>
>   I waive the zusetum of the sin;
>   The hazard of concealing;
>   But oh! It hardens a' within.
>   And petrifies the feeling.

Your friends, and you too, very probably, would wish you to settle respectably—in something like the style to which you have been accustomed at home; and therefore, forsooth, you are to wait, no one knows how long. But if you look back only a generation or two, you will very probably find that some of your ancestors began life in a very humble fashion. Now it is by no means certain that they were less happy than then when they afterwards occupied a much higher position; and I maintain that *happiness* is what is **most desirable,** also that it is inseparable from virtue, and that it is not nearly so difficult of attainment **as** many imagine.

"Death is the of **gate** life." When, therefore we leave this world our more real life then **first begins. And, without doubt, it is for this end that we are placed here, in a preparatory state,** where we have ample opportunity of acquiring heavenly habits. Now, mark and see for yourself among your acquaintance whether it is not the most orderly, married people, with families—those who are in the habitual endeavour to fulfill God's holy laws— that are in the enjoyment of the greatest amount of real happiness. I by no means assert that they are so riotuously joyous as the dissolute. The joys of the latter are merely transient, and soon give place to sorrow and remorse, or lead them on to ruin ; while the joys of the former, partaking of the nature of Him from whom they spring, will doubtless go on increasing to eternity.

But I must come to a pause; the few pages to which I have limited myself will not permit me to do anything like full justice to my subject. I trust, however, that I have said enough to put some young persons who may be lead to read these remarks so far on their guard as to *prevent* them from entering on a path which to all is dangerous, to very many fatal. In reference to all the numerous phases of this evil it may, with the greatest emphasis, be declared that " Prevention is better than cure."

CHAPTER X.

A SPECIAL CHAPTER FOR YOUNG **WOMEN.**

Advice upon this subject is very much needed. I am assured that it is a subject not often **talked** of in families—at least as it ought to be ; nor is it much alluded to in the pulpit; and the result is that young people commonly get their notions about it from those only a little older than themselves, and who therefore know but little more than they do; or from those who form their opinions from the abuse they see of it, and so hold degrading and unworthy ideas respecting it. Sometimes all that is known about it amounts to this—that it is a delightful thing to be married.

It is quite true that it often is, and always ought to be, delightful; still, you know, it is frequently quite the reverse. You cannot then be too cautious in the matter.

Nothing can be more orderly, right, proper, and holy than marriage. It is not, however, quite so simple an affair as you may fancy. Every good thing—and this is one of the best—requires some effort to obtain it; and unless you take the right course you must not expect to succeed.

You may often see a young woman who, from not entertaining correct views on the point, is certainly taking a wrong course; her endeavors being rather to make what she considers a good match, than, by acquiring kind and orderly habits, to qualify herself to become worthy of a worthy husband.

That the best things are liable to the greatest abuses is notorious; and from the lamentable fact that marriage is often abused, we may fairly infer its pre-eminent worth. In truth there is nothing more valuable. It is then highly injurious to entertain low notions respecting it; and men who indulge in loose conversation on the subject are likely, at the same time to think meanly of women. Beware of them; and if you hear them expressing such opinions in your presence, withdraw from them at once as unworthy of your company. Never fear but they will respect you the more for the rebuke.

Of course, you are looking forward to settle happily, and will do your best for that purpose. On this let me remark that all happiness—that is, all that is genuine, and therefore worthy of the name—comes from connection with the One great source of all good; and He has freely and fully provided all the means necessary for our being happy, both here and hereafter. He has placed each of us where it is best for us to be, and in the circumstances that are best for us at the time; and this applies to you and to me now. How much soever appearances may be to the contrary, He cares as much for each of us as if we were the sole objects of His care. It is only by doing our duty, in humble dependence on His assistance, which He never withholds, that we can be happy. It behoves you then to consider well what is your duty, in order that you may do it, and may enjoy the blessings He is so ready to bestow. I hope you have been a loving and dutiful daughter, an affectionate sister and a faithful friend : then you may have good ground of hope for the future.

When a prospect of marriage occurs, you cannot do better than consult your mother, aunt, or other discreet relative that has your welfare at heart, from whom you may reasonably expect the best and most disinterested advice; and this it will be well for you to be guided by. Women of mature years can judge far better than you whether a man is likely to make a good husband. You should likewise quietly and cautiously make your own observations among your married acquaintance, especially where you believe there is a comfortable and happy home. You will doubtless find that, to a very great extent, this happy home depends on the wife's management and economy. Very often it happens that, where two husbands have the same income, with the same number of children, there will be comfort in the one home and discomfort in the other. Now there must be a reason for this; and you should endeavor to find it out, and profit by the lesson. It is said, 'Cleanliness is next to godliness;' and truly the value of cleanliness cannot be overrated. In point of time it should go before godliness; for where there is not cleanliness there can hardly be godliness; and the health of body and mind are greatly dependent on these two. Moreover, where can there be complete happiness without health ?

One of the most prolific sources of matrimonial difficulties is the lack of knowledge on the part of wives of the duties of housekeeping. In these days there are a hundred young ladies who can drum on the piano to one who can make a good loaf of bread. Yet a hungry husband cares more for a good dinner than he does —as long as his appetite is unappeased—to listen to the music of the spheres. Heavy bread has made many heavy hearts, given rise to dyspepsia—horrid dyspepsia—and its herd of accompanying torments. Girls who desire that their husbands should be amiable and kind, should learn how to make good bread. When a young man is courting, he can live well at home; or, if he has to go a distance to pay his addresses, he usually obtains good meals at a hotel or an eating house; but when he is married and gets to housekeeping, his wife assumes the functions of his mother or his landlord, and it is fortunate for her her if she has been educated so as to know what a good table is. Those who are entirely dependent upon hired cooks make a very poor show at housekeeping. The stomach performs a very important part in the economy of humanity, and wives who are forgetful of this fact commit a serious mistake.

You know full well that most young men—and most young women too—are desirous of marrying and having a family; but they do not sufficiently consider that it is God who gives them this desire, and that for the wisest of purposes; not only that this world may be peopled, but also that its inhabitants may be prepared for heaven.

Nothing is more certain than that marriage affords the fairest opportunities for preparing for a better world. In it we have others dearer than ourselves to think about and provide for; and in doing so, we have often to practise that very useful virtue—self-denial. Let me here impress upon you most deeply, that it is only by making others happy that we can become happy ourselves. The angels, we may be assured, are happy, because they are always actively good; and for a similar reason it is that God Himself is infinitely happy. If you try to secure your own happiness by any other means than a faithful discharge of your duty to God and your neighbor, you will certainly and deservedly fail.

I dare say you find that young men are fond of your company and of paying you every polite attention, and you, as a right-minded woman, are well pleased to be so treated. It is due to you *as a woman*. Now each of them is—or ought to be—looking out for a wife; and it is well that you should know this. It is, too, more important than you perhaps are aware that you should be carefully making your own observations, so that, when the time arrives for one of them to ask you to become his wife, you may not be taken by surprise, but may know how to act on the occasion.

Let me here caution you against a failing that is common among young women; I mean that of making themselves too cheap. They feel flattered by the attentions paid to them, and are not sufficiently aware that many young men are fond of indulging in flattery; and such, if they find a young woman weak enough to be pleased with it, will perhaps play upon her feelings and gain her affections, without having any honorable intentions towards her.

As a protection against such, I recommend you to have a proper respect for yourself, and to consider with what object or purpose you receive their attentions. If you respond without an object, you may be doing them wrong; if you accept them when they have no right intentions, you allow them to wrong you. For this purpose consider well what you are—a human being intended for an eternity of bliss. God has made you a WOMAN; and, believe me, as there is no fairer so there is no nobler creature than woman. She is formed to be her husband's help-mate and the mother of his children; and the all-important work of training these for heaven depends mainly upon her. Great, then, is her responsibility; but God has given her the requisite love and power to do her duty with satisfaction and delight. He has placed you in this beautiful world that by doing your duty as a daughter, sister, wife, mother and friend, you may become fitted to enter His heavenly kingdom.

During your courtship let me entreat you to be very careful and circumspect. There is no period in life that can compare with this delightful season. It is or should be, full of sunshine and sparkling with the poetry of life; but alas! to many it is the opposite. A want of judgment—a momentary indiscretion, has not only blotted out this beautiful spring-time of life, but has marred, darkened and blighted the whole of the after life time.

No maiden can, under any circumstance, place her character in the hands of any man before marriage. No matter how sincere the love, how ardent the protestations, how earnest or plausable the pleadings, you must not, you can not surrender your honor. You must preserve your prudence and virtue, it is only by the possession of these, that you can keep the love and respect of your lover. Be firm, be circumspect, a rash word or a false step may extinguish forever all your bright hopes and prospective joys. Even should your lover redeem his promises and take you to be his wife, this indiscretion or crime will surely hang over you like a curse, creating discord, trouble and sorrow, the greatest portion of which will fall to your share.

You must know that young men, however amiable, worthy or honorable they may be, **may** in a moment of intense excitement, **commit a sin, that in their calmer moments they would not be guilty of for worlds.**

But under all circumstances, you will be looked upon **to resist any advances and** maintain your purity and virtue. No matter how high the tide of passion may run in unguarded moments and set in against heaven and against society, the terrible and painful ebb will surely follow and leave you stranded forever on the bleak and barren shore of your earthly existence.

There is no state of life more honorable, useful and happy, than **that of a wife and mother.** There must and ever will be inequalities **of station, but happiness is equally** attainable in them all. **To be happy,** however, **you must** be good; of course, I do not **mean absolutely** good; **for** 'there is none good but One ;' but **I** mean that you should be relatively good, and should aim at becoming better and more innocent as you advance in life. Now you cannot respect yourself unless you **know that you are worthy** of respect; and if you **do not respect** yourself, you cannot expect that anybody else will; **and in** such case you will not be worthy **of the love of any good man, and** none such will be likely to pay **court to you.** If, however, **you take the right means, in** which **I** include prayer for divine guidance, you will have the respect and friendship of all your **acquaintance;** and then in **God's own** time **and, let me** add, without your seeking it, **the man whom you can make happy,** and who can make you happy, **will** present himself **and propose to make you his** wife, **if it** be **God's will that** you **should become one.**

Here are **two** very important points for your consideration; first that it should be **your** constant endeavor to make your husband happy; and, second, **that,** before you consent to marry him, you should ascertain that he has those qualifications that will secure **your** happiness. It most nearly concerns **yourself that you do your duty to God and your** neighbor **at all times, so that** it becomes **your habit: and you** will find **it much easier,** and safer too, **to do it every day rather than only on particular occasions; for this** would require **a special effort,** and for the time, perhaps, put **you** into a state of excitement, **which, in** all probability, would be succeeded by a depression **of spirits.** What you should rather aim at is a uniformly cheerful state of mind resulting from a conscious and confident dependence on Providence. If your husband knows from experience that such is your character he cannot fail, provided he be worthy of you, to be content and happy.

It is the nature of young women to be affectionate, and it is pleasant and usual for them to have several dear friends enjoying more or less of their confidence. Among these may be included some of their male acquaintance. Now, while they may esteem each of these as they would a dear cousin, they should know and act upon the knowledge, that it is only to one they can give their unlimited confidence and undivided affection as a wife. It is the height of cruelty and wickedness for either a man or a woman to trifle with another's affection. Such base conduct has cost many a young woman her health and peace, and even her life, and cannot therefore be too much deprecated and avoided.

Let me then advise you to be very cautious before you allow a young man to pay you such marked attentions as may lead to marriage. It is not, you know, to terminate in seven years, like an apprenticeship or a commercial partnership, but it is an engagement for the life of one of the parties. I want you then to profit by the experience of others, too many of whom enter into marriage from light and low considerations; and not to settle in life till you, and also your friends, see that there is a reasonable prospect of your securing happiness, as well as comfort and a respectable position.

When a young woman has property, or expects it, or is possessed of superior personal attractions, she should be especially prudent in her conduct towards the numerous admirers which such qualifications usually attract. No woman should allow herself to accept the attentions of any man who does not possess those sterling qualities which will command her respect, or whose love is directed to her fortune or beauty rather than herself. On such a one she can place no reliance; for, should illness or misfortune overtake her, she may find herself deprived of that love which she had valued as the great treasure of her life. Possessed of this, she feels that earthly riches are but of secondary importance, and that the want of them can never make her poor.

Moreover, a worthier man than any of her interested suitors, may have a sincere respect and affection for her, but be kept in the background by the over-zealous attention of his rivals. Still if she has sufficient self-command to patiently and calmly investigate their general private character, she may find reason to decline their suit, and may discover that the more modest and retiring youth is the one that is deserving of her love.

While on this subject, let me caution you against the foolish affection which some girls practise in order to attract the attention of young men. In their company, be natural in your manners, open and friendly and ready to converse on general subjects; not appearing to expect that every one who pays you the ordinary courtesies of society is going to fall in love with you. This mode of behavior, which is more common with those who are vain of their beauty than with others, frequently leads to such young women being more neglected than their less pretending sisters; for prudent young men, who are impressed with the necessity of a right decision in the all important step of marriage, instinctively shrink from those who seem unwilling to give them a fair opportunity of judging whether their hearts and minds are as attractive as their persons.

You may innocently admire many a young man for the noble qualities God has bestowed upon him, without at all entertaining the idea either that he would make you happy as his wife, or you him as your husband. Thank God, we are constituted of such different temperaments that all may find suitable partners without clashing with others' tastes, if they will only be content to watch and wait.

It is the part of a young man to *watch*, to be actively desirous of meeting with a suitable partner. In doing this his first consideration should be to seek for such a one as he can make happy; not to look primarily for beauty, fortune, wit, or accomplishments —things all very good in themselves, but by no means constituting the essentials of happiness. If he is influenced by pure and simple motives, he will not find or expect to find, more than one that can satisfy his desire; and he will not be in much danger of exciting the envy or the rivalry of his companions.

On the other hand, it is becoming in a young woman to *wait* patiently, till, from the assidnous and respectful attentions of a young man, she can have no doubt that he is in earnest ; when, and not before, she may freely give him her company, and with every expectation of a happy result. Be assured that no sensible young man is ever attracted by a young woman whom he sees on the lookout for a lover; he is more likely to think meanly of her, and to avoid her society.

It may, however, happen that a young man makes the offer before the young woman knows enough of him for it to be right for her to accept it, and before he on his part ought to take the step. In such case it would be well for her, even supposing she is inclined to like him, to tell him that he has taken her by surprise, and that she cannot think of entering on so important a subject without consulting her friends, to whom she accordingly refers him. It would then become her duty to intimate to him that, although his attentions are agreeable to them, he must wait a while, till, from further acquaintance, they are enabled to judge whether it will conduce to the mutual happiness of their daughter and himself for her to accept the offer he has so kindly made.

But it is not only young men who are apt to be hasty in these matters: it is, as is well known, not uncommon for parents, especially mothers, very soon after a young man has begun to pay attention to their daughter, to give him to understand that they wish to know his intentions in reference to her. By such proceedings a young man may be taken aback, and either hurry into a match which turns out unhappily, or be led to withdraw from a union which might have resulted in the happiness of all the parties concerned.

That your parents should wish you to be married, is only natural, especially if their own marriage has been a happy one. It will be gratifying to them to see a worthy young man paying attention to you, and, most probably, they will let things take their own course. Marriage is too important a matter to admit of being hastened.

There are, I am aware, unwise parents who, from various motives, will throw obstacles in the way of young people who are desirous of coming together. Some are so selfish as to be unwilling to part with their daughter, preferring their own happiness to hers. Others are so silly as to think no ordinary man good enough for her, and therefore, if they had their own way, would leave her to become an old maid. Fortunately, such short-sighted people are not unfrequently outwitted.

If your parents are—as I hope they are—reasonable in their views and expectations, one of the chief concerns of their life will be the promotion of your happiness; and it behoves you to pay the utmost deference to their opinion; and should they, from circumstances they become aware of, deem it advisable that you should either postpone or even break off an engagement, they will, doubtless, give you such weighty reasons as will justify you in acting on their advice. Where, however, as sometimes happens, they unwisely refuse their consent to their child's marriage, at a time when she well knows, from her own feelings, and also from the sanction she receives from the opinion of trustworthy and judicious friends, that she would be making a real sacrifice were she to comply with their wishes,—if, I say, under such circumstances, she acts disobediently and marries the man she loves, more blame attaches to the parents than to herself; and the sooner they forgive her the better.

It is very common for young men, when going into the company of young women, together with their best dress to put on their best behavior : in fact, to assume a character which is not their natural one, but far superior to it. Some hold the opinion that 'All is fair in love and war.' To me it appears there cannot be greater folly and wickedness than for young people who are thinking of marrying to attempt to deceive each other. What is the good of it? A very short period of married life will entirely dispel the illusion. I suppose people of the world may think it fair to overreach one another in their dealings, saying, 'Everyone for himself.' They have no intention of seeking to promote the other's happiness: present gain is all they want. But a married pair, to be happy, must respect and esteem, as well as love, each other; and this cannot be attained except by the constant endeavor to be as well as to *appear* true and good.

That young men should behave well in the presence of women is only natural and right. None but a fool would do otherwise. But you, long before thinking of marrying, should take all fair means to learn what are the general conduct and habits of your male acquaintance, in their family circle and with their daily connections. Are they good-humored and kind—able to bear the troubles they meet with? are they industrious, frugal, temperate, religious, chaste? Have they had the prudence to insure against sickness and death? or, on the other **hand, are** they addicted to drinking, smoking, betting, keeping late hours, frequenting **casinos**, &c.? Your mother and other prudent friends will assist **you** to find this out. Those **who do not come up to** the proper standard, **however agreeable they may be as acquaintance, certainly cannot make good husbands. In company of such, it behoves you to be well on your** guard, and **accept no attention from them.** Should you marry such a one, you would be sure **to be miserable.**

While, however, it is **quite right that you** should be **careful about the character of the young man who is** paying court to you, **it is of far** more importance to you that **you should be careful** about your own, and this whether you marry or not. **Indeed,** a chief object in our being placed in this world is that we **may acquire** good habits, and so be fitted to associate with 'the just made **perfect in heaven.'**

Be **very guarded in your actions and demeanor. Cultivate purity of** heart and thought. **No woman is fit to become a wife who is** not perfectly modest in **word, deed and thought. No young** man, who is worth having, **would ever entertain the thought for a moment of taking the girl for a wife who is habitually careless in her conversation and displays a levity in her manners.** Young men **may like** your free **and hearty girls to laugh and talk** with, but as to taking one for a wife, let me **assure you they** would not tolerate the idea for a moment.

You **may at times be** unavoidably compelled **to hear a** vulgar word spoken, or an indelicate illusion made: in every instance maintain a rigid insensibility. It **is not** enough that you cast **down your** eyes or turn your head, you must act as if you did not **hear it; appear as** if you did not comprehend it. You **ought to receive no more impression from** remarks or illusions **of this** character **than a block of wood. Unless you maintain this standing, and preserve this high-toned purity of manner, you will be greatly depreciated in the opinion of all** men whose opinion **is** worth having, and you deprive yourself **of much** influence and respect which it is your privilege to possess and exert.

Courtship, after all, is a momentous matter. After **taking all the** counsel that may be offered, you must at last, in a great measure, rely on your own judgment. Within a few short months you have to decide, from what you can see of a man, whether you will have him, in preference to your parents, friends, and all others that you know, to be a life companion. What can you do? How shall you judge? How arrive at a correct conclusion? My dear young girl, there is only One who can assist you. He in His mercy to your helplessness and weakness, has given to every virtuous and pure-minded woman a wonderful, mysterious and subtle instinct; a peculiar faculty that cannot be analyzed by reason, a faculty that men do not possess, and one in which they do not generally believe. At this all important period, this eventful crisis in your life, this womanly instinct guides and saves you. You can feel in a moment the presence or influence of a base, sensual and unworthy nature. An electric-like thrill animates you, and you are naturally repulsed from him. When your suitor is a man of incongruous temper, ungenial habits, and of a morose and unsympathetic disposition, this same precious, divine instinct acts, and the man feels, though he cannot tell why, that all his arts and aspirations are in vain; it will seldom be necessary for you to tell him verbally of his failure; but should such a one blindly insist upon intruding his attentions, do not hesitate to tell him kindly but firmly your decision. Should your suitor be one who is worthy, who will make you happy, this same blessed instinct will whisper in your soul the happy news. From the first interview there is frequently thrown around the maiden a peculiar, undefined spell; she will feel differently in his presence, and watch him with other eyes than she has for the rest of men, and in due time, when he shall ask her to decide upon the question which shall seal the temporal and eternal destiny of two human souls, she will gladly respond, giving in loving trustfulness that which is the most precious, the most enviable thing on earth:—a maiden's heart, a woman's love.

Many persons of both sexes, however amiable and pure their minds may be, should conscientiously abstain from marriage. This applies to all who have a tendency to consumption, scrofula, insanity or any other of those diseases which are so frequently transmitted to offspring. This very important matter is not sufficiently known, and therefore is not attended to as it ought to be; hence the great amount of sickness and early death among children.

The tendency to inherit qualities is very evident in the case of drunkards, whose children are often inclined to practise the vice

of their parents. The children of the blind and of the deaf and
dumb are also liable to be afflicted as their parents were. These
facts go far to show that it is literally true that the sins of the
fathers are visited upon the children. It is, however, gratifying
to know—and there are many well-attested cases to prove it—
that, whereas the children born to a man while he was addicted
to drunkenness were similarly addicted to that vice, those born
after he gave up his vicious indulgence, and by that means improved his bodily health, were free from the evil tendency.

One strong reason why near relations should not intermarry is
that, as the same general tendencies prevail in families, when the
parents are nearly related, they are very likely to have the same evil
tendency, whatever that may be; and, therefore, there is a great
probability that their children will also have the same, but more
strongly developed; and, consequently, the difficulty of their
overcoming it will be much increased.

How plainly then is it the duty of those about to marry, as well
as of those who are married, to strive to their utmost, with God's
help, to overcome disorderly habits of every kind; for, be assured,
it is only by such means they can hope to be blessed with good
and healthy children, and thereby contribute to their own happiness, and at the same time to the improvement of the race as subjects both of this world and of heaven.

As it is by no means certain that you will marry, and the time
may come when it will no longer be convenient to your parents
to support you, it will be good for you, keeping these contingen-
cies in mind, to qualify yourself to earn your own maintenance
by some honest industry. You will then have a right feeling of
independence, and not be tempted to marry, as too many young
women do, not from the true principle of sincere affection, but
mainly for a living. They may thus obtain a competency, and
jog on comfortably; but they have no right to expect that genuine happiness which I recommend you to aim at. When, too,
you see so many left widows, with small families, and, as we say,
totally unprovided for, you will become sensible of the soundness
of the advice I am offering you. As the Lord's tender mercies
are over all His works, it is evident, from what is occurring around
us, that trouble and adversity are better suited to the state of some
people, to prepare them for their eternal destination, than any

amount of prosperity would be. The poor are no less at children than the rich, and He cares equally, that is, infinitely, for them all. It is certainly wise, then, to be prepared to meet adversity, should He suffer it to come upon you.

Again, suppose you should not have any suitable offer of marriage, such as you would feel it your duty to accept, you are not on that account to be disheartened, and fancy yourself overlooked by Providence. Single life is evidently the best for some persons : they escape many troubles which perhaps they would find it very hard to bear. There are many ways in which single people can lead a useful life, and be as happy as the day is long. No one that is actively useful can be unhappy. What do you see around you ? Many, I admit, who are not so happy as we should like them to be; but in most cases, if we could fully investigate the matter, it would perhaps be found to have arisen from their thinking too much about themselves and not enough for others. But, on the other hand, it not unfrequently happens, when a woman is left, and sees that the support and welfare of herself and her children depend on her own exertions, she is enabled so successfully to put forth her energies, and to employ her talents which, till she needed them, she hardly knew she possessed, as to surprise both herself and the most sanguine of her friends.

Now, it must be confessed that we are fallen creatures, and therefore prone to evil. We are consequently always in danger of going wrong and forming bad habits; but our heavenly Father watches over us at all times, and gives us power 'to refuse the evil and choose the good.' We are, I know full well, too much inclined to yield to evil influences; still, as we always have divine aid if we implore it, I am not sure that, on the whole, it is not as easy to acquire good habits as bad ones. This much is certain, that whichever we acquire—good or bad—they are likely to remain with us; and are not easily to be got rid of.

Among the subjects deserving attention, as affecting our happiness, is one on which perhaps I am not entitled to say much. I refer to dress. Now, I hold it to be a duty for people to dress well, that is, according to their position, means, and age; and this not so much for their own sakes as for the sake of giving pleasure to others. It is, I admit, difficult to determine how much of one's income should be devoted to dress; but I think few will deny that, at present, dress occupies too much time, attention and money. For my own part, I confess, I am most affected by female dress; and although certainly I **like to** see women well dressed, and would rather see them a little too fine than slovenly, I am often pained at witnessing the extravagance and, to me, rid- **iculous taste exhibited.** Whenever I see a **handsome and** expen- sive dress trailing **in the** dirt, **I regard it as** culpable waste and in bad taste; and when I see it **accidentally** trodden **on, I am not** sorry. I am inclined to believe that many **women can hardly** find time or opportunity to perform any useful duty: they have quite as much as they, poor things, can do, to take care of their **dress.** I also believe—and this is the serious point of the matter —that many a young man is deterred from soliciting a maiden in marriage, by knowing that his means would not enable him to let her dress as he is accustomed to see her; and this is doubtless **one of the many reasons why so many of both** sexes remain un- **married. I hold, too, that whatever forms an obstacle to mar-** riage has a tendency, at the **same time, to obstruct the entrance** to heaven.

I will now allude to some of the duties which will involve upon **you as a wife; and recollect that it** is on the faithful discharge of **these duties that your** happiness, **here and** hereafter, **mainly de-** pends. All labor is honorable, and you know who it is that **says, you** 'My Father worketh hitherto, and I work.' Being married, **you** must make your husband feel, 'There is no place like home.' His business will probably take him from home most of the day; and it should be your care—as I doubt not it will be your delight— to see to his comfort, both before he starts and when he returns. It may sometimes happen, in his fighting the battle of life, that he has to encounter much that is unpleasant, and he may return home depressed. You will then have to **cheer him; and be as-** sured, **no one can** do it so **effectually, so pleasantly, aye, and so** easily, as yourself.

It is not to sweep the house, and make the bed, and darn the socks, and cook the meals, chiefly, that a man wants a wife. If this is all he needs, hired help can do it cheaper than a wife. If this is all, when a young man calls to see a young lady, send him **into** the pantry to taste the bread and cake she has made. Send him to inspect the needle-work and bed-making; or put a broom into her hands, and send him to witness its use. Such things are important and the wise young man will quietly look after them. But what a true man most wants of a true wife is her companionship, sympathy, courage, and love. The way of life has many dreary places in it, and a man needs a companion to go with him. A man is sometimes overtaken with misfortune; he meets with failure and defeat; trials and temptations beset him; and he needs one to stand by and sympathize. He has some stern battles to fight with poverty, with enemies, and with sin; and he needs a woman that, while he puts his arm around her and feels that he has something to fight for, will help him fight; that will put her lips to his ear and whisper words of counsel, and her hands to his heart and impart new inspirations. All through life—through storm and through sunshine, conflict and victory, and through adverse and favoring winds—man needs a woman's love. The heart yearns for it. A sister's or a mother's love will hardly supply the need. Yet many seek for nothing further than success in housework. Justly enough, half of these get nothing more; the other half, surprised beyond measure, have got more than they sought. Their wives surprise them by bringing a nobler idea of marriage, and disclosing a treasury of courage, sympathy and love.

And I would here caution you against giving way to little misunderstandings in early married life. Sometimes trifling matters for want of some forbearance or concession on one side or the other, perhaps on both sides, accumulate into serious results. These differences might be avoided by married partners studying each other's peculiarities of character, with the aim of mutually correcting, in a kindly spirit, any wrong tendency or temper which may sometimes show itself. Should you find you have inadvertently given pain or uneasiness to your husband, do not rest until you have ascertained the cause of his disquiet, and succeed in allaying the unhappy feeling. The earnest desire to please each other should by no means terminate on the wedding day, but as studiously continued through married life. Each should always endeavor to think the best of the other, and instantly reject every thought that might tend to weaken the bond of mutual preference and perfect trust.

If he be wise, he will leave the housekeeping entirely to you;

his time and attention can be better employed elsewhere. To
enable you to do this wisely, you should, long before you marry,
become familiar with the quality and prices of articles of consumption, and where they can be best obtained. Every wife
should be able to cook well, whether she has to do it herself or
not. Health and good humor greatly depend upon the food's
being of good quality, well cooked, and nicely served up. She
should also be able, if needful, to make and mend her own and
children's clothes.

Too much importance cannot be attached to cleanliness. Men
may be careless as to their own personal appearance, and may,
from the nature of their business, be negligent in their dress,
but they dislike to see any disregard in the dress and appearance
of their wives. Nothing so depresses a man and makes him dislike and neglect his home as to have a wife who is slovenly in
her dress and unclean in her habits. Beauty of face and form
will not compensate for these defects; the charm of purity and
cleanliness never ends but with life itself. These are matters
that do not involve any great labor or expense. The use of the
bath, and the simplest fabrics, shaped by your own supple fingers,
will be all that is necessary. These attractions will act like a
magnet upon your husband. Never fear that there will be any
influence strong enough to take him from your side.

An experience of many years of observation has convinced me
that where a pure, industrious and cheerful wife meets her husband with a bright smile on the threshold of her dwelling, that
man will never leave her home for any other place.

As all people are liable to illness, every young woman should
aim at being an efficient nurse. In case of illness, it is now generally admitted that good nursing is of more value than medicine.
To a sick husband, a little gruel or other trifle prepared and given
by wife's own hand will confer much more benefit than if prepared and given by another. Should it happen to you to fall ill,
you may expect your husband will do his best; but you must not
be surprised if he is not your equal in that department. Nursing
is one of the many useful things which women can do better than
men. A practical knowledge of nursing will enable you to be
useful beyond your own family, and will enhance your value as a
neighbor.

You have often, I trust, experienced the pleasure of serving others from disinterested motives, and found that the pleasure has been deeper and purer when you have engaged in doing good to those who could not make you any return. This you have found to be the case whenever you have had charge of a baby— one of those little ones of whom the Lord says: 'Their angels do always behold the face of my Father who is in Heaven.' You have perhaps been surprised to find how easy it was to perform such a duty; and let me assure you that you may always expect to find it easy to perform your duty in that state of life to which it shall please God to call you. He never requires anything from any of his creatures beyond what He gives them power to do. He is no hard task-master. You have only to look to Him, and do your best, and then you may safely leave the result in His hands. Our Lord, you know, says, 'My yoke is easy, and my burden is light.'

Of all God's creatures, I know no happier one than a young mother with a good husband and a healthy baby. I say a *healthy* baby, for that implies healthy parents, especially a healthy mother. She may justly feel proud that God has intrusted a young immortal to her care, and she should at all times bear in mind that it is His gift. While it is on all hands considered honorable to hold a commission from the President and to fill a high office, contributing to the welfare of many people, a mother may feel her office, at least, as honorable, seeing she has entrusted to her the rearing and training of an immortal being, and that she holds her commission direct from the King of kings. For, recollect, it is only by God's blessing that she becomes a mother; for such is the present state of society that many very worthy married people have not the privilege of offspring, although they are intensely fond of children, and seem to have no other earthly want. They may nevertheless be very useful and therefore, happy in a different sphere, by the adoption of nephews and nieces, or in some similar way.

At the birth of her first child, there is opened in the mother's heart a new well of love, such as she had not known before: and although she may fancy that this is all spent upon her babe, it is not so; for she loves her God, her husband, and everybody else better than ever. The father too, is similarly affected: he also has a warmer love for his wife and for all his connections.

A similar idea is well expressed by Möhler, a German writer, who says:—' The power of selfishness, which is inwoven with our whole being, is altogether broken by marriage; and, **by degrees, love,** becoming more and more pure, takes its place. **When a** man marries, he gives himself up entirely to *another* being: **in** this affair of life he first goes out of himself, and inflicts the first deadly wound on his egotism. By every child with which his marriage is blessed, Nature renews the same attack on **his self-** hood; causes him to live less for himself, and more—even without being distinctly conscious of it—for others: his heart expands in proportion as the claimants upon it increase; and, bursting the **bonds of its former** narrow exclusiveness, it eventually extends its sympathies to all around.'

Whenever a mother is supplying her baby with the food which God has so wisely provided for it, or is ministering to any other **of its numerous and increasing** wants, she may feel that everything she does for it is pleasing **to her heavenly Father, and** has its immediate reward in the delight she **experiences in the act.**

I can fancy that, when a mother has washed **her baby, and,** before she dresses it, has a good romp with it, smothering it **with** kisses, calling it all the beauties and darlings and pets and jewels she can think of, and talking any amount of nonsense at the **top** of her voice—the baby all the while cooing, chirping, or **even** screaming with delight; at such a time, I say, I can easily **fancy** that the angels are looking on approvingly and enjoying the **scene. And why not?** ' Of such is the Kingdom of Heaven.'

From the time that an infant first becomes conscious of its wants, and long afterwards, it looks to its mother to supply them all, fully believing her able to do it. She is, in fact, in place of God to it: and it would be well for many of us if we trusted our heavenly Father as simply and as fully as the infant does **its earthly** mother.

Those who know no better, when they see a mother patiently watching her sleeping babe, **might wonder** that she does not feel the want of company. She has, however, company that they know not of, and of which even she herself may not be conscious. If only our eyes were open, we might see that she is not the only one that is so engaged—that angels are also occupied in watching the babe and in supporting her. I entirely agree with

Dr. Watts, where, in his ' Cradle Hymn,' he makes the mother say:—

> Hush ! my babe, lie still and slumber,
> Holy angels guard thy bed !

You probably know the beautiful Irish superstition that, when a baby smiles in its sleep, the angels are whispering to it.

Before I became a father, I took little or no interest in babies ; I rather thought them troublesome things. But the arrival of one of my own wrought a great change in me. It enlarged at once my views and my heart, and I had higher and stronger motives to exertion. My interest in them had not yet begun to werken; and I have no reason to think it ever will.

Girls are differently constituted from boys. God makes the intellect predominate in males, and affection in females. Accordingly, a little girl early shows a love for a doll, regarding it quite as her baby, and never taking into account that is not alive. She has many of a mother's cares and anxieties, as well as pleasures about it, indeed as many as she is then capable of. It is a constant source of amusement and employment to her. In all this we may plainly see the hand of Providence: it forms a suitable introduction to some of the interesting and important duties which will devolve on her if it should be His good pleasure for her to become a mother.

The other day I met a group of four or five little girls, the principal one, some nine years old, very carefully carrying a baby. On my saying to her, 'You seem almost as pleased as if it were your own baby,' she gave me an innocent smile, and said—rather proudly, I thought—'It is my own, please, sir.' I took it she was the sister, and not a hired nurse.

You will, I dare say, readily see the object I now have in view. It is that I wish to impress on you how desirable it is that you should take every opportunity of becoming acquainted with the habits and wants of babies, and the best way of managing them. The more you have to do with them the more you will like the labor, and the easier and more delightful it will become. It is fair that, before you have children of your own, you should get your knowledge as to the management of them, by experience with other people's. I take it for granted you will at all times do your best for them. You will then have but little cause to fear accident; and if accident should happen—as with all your care it sometimes will—you will have more confidence in your powers, and will be more likely to do what is best at the moment, than if you were unused to children. Much of the disease and early death that happen among children arises from the ignorance of the mothers; who, however, are often much more to be pitied than blamed in the matter. They had never been properly taught their duties towards their future offspring.

It will be very advantageous to you, to procure a copy of a very valuable work called "*Our Own Family Doctor.*"*

It contains a vast amount of valuable information respecting health, disease and other kindred subjects, written in so plain a style that simple people cannot fail to understand it. The volume I consider so suitable to young women about to marry, that parents should not hesitate to place it in their hands. I would especially mention the chapters entitled " Women and their Diseases," " Children and their Care," "Accidents and Emergencies," and the chapter to the youth of both sexes.

These portions of the work alone are worth tenfold more than the price asked for the whole work. I am certain they are calculated to save the lives of many children and not a few mothers.

Few mothers are, perhaps, sufficiently aware of the great influence which their manners, habits and conversation have upon the tender minds of their children, even from birth. The child should grow up with a feeling of reverence for its parents, which can only be the case when wisdom as well as affection is exercised in its bringing up. Hence the necessity of the mother's fitting herself, both *intellectually* and *morally*, for her sacred office, that the child may become accustomed to yield perfect obedience to her wishes from a principle of love, and may acquire, as it advances in life. the habit of yielding a like obedience to that which is right.

---

* "*Our Own Family Doctor*," and complete medical adviser, containing every known fact that can promote health, cure disease and prolong life, with a careful analysis of everything relating to courtship and marriage and the production, management and bringing up of healthy families. Illustrated with 134 Engravings, 604 pages, octavo, English Cloth, Beveled Boards. Price, $3.00.

As you well know that you are not perfect yourself, you must be prepared to find that your husband has also his imperfections; and it is no unimportant **part of your duty to** help him to get rid of them. Indeed it is one **of the highest uses** of marriage for each partner to assist the other on the journey to the heavenly Canaan. But, before you attempt to point out a fault in him, consider how you had best proceed, so as to attain your object; for, unless you adopt a judicious mode, and an affectionate as well as an earnest manner, you may do as much harm as good. You must also carefully watch your opportunity; for what would be favorably received at **one** time, **and under certain circumstances, might, under other circumstances, give offence, and altogether fail of the good effect intended** and hoped for. You do not **know how powerful you may be for** good to your husband. **There is much truth in the saying,** 'A man is what a woman **makes him.'**

Respecting the good influence of virtuous love, Tennyson says:—

> For indeed I know
> Of no more subtle **master** under heaven
> Than is the maiden passion for a maid,
> Not only to keep down the base in man,
> But teach him thought, and amiable words,
> And courtliness, and the desire of fame,
> And love of truth, and all that makes a man.

Previous to your marriage, it will be expedient for you not to **give your lover that full and unlimited** confidence which it will **be your duty—and your inclination,** too—to give him when he **becomes your husband.** I refer chiefly to family and other private **matters, not to anything he ought to know to** enable him to judge of your character and **position.** Many unhappy marriages have been brought **about through the** young woman's letting it be known that she has **'great expectations.'** A worthless fellow may, in consequence, **have succeeded in winning her hand.**

There is another point to which I must just allude before concluding **this address.** It is doubtless the order of **Providence for** marriages to take place, **when possible,** on our arriving at years of maturity. But I would **guard** you against the evil results of *too early* marriages, before either body or mind is perfectly matured. We scarcely need consult either medical or moral science to satisfy ourselves on this by no. means trifling point. We may find in society too many sad instances of such immature and indiscreet unions. The minds of young persons should be expanded by a certain amount of experience in the world before entering upon engagements involving so many momentous duties.

In your daily walks abroad, if you examine the countenances of those you meet, you will doubtless be led to conclude that there is a great deal of disease and misery in the world; but, judging from my own observation, I think you will find that the greater number of persons exhibit signs of health and happiness. Much of the disease and misery with which the world is afflicted, is the direct result of the misconduct of the individuals themselves; but no little of it is attributable to their parents, who have neglected or violated God's laws of health, their misconduct thus affecting their descendants ' to the third and fourth generation.' I cannot therefore, too much impress upon you the importance of your honestly trying to find out any bad habits to which you are inclined, with a view to getting rid of them, one by one, and supplying their place by good habits. By pursuing this course, you will not only do much for your own happiness, but also for that of your children, if God should bless you with a family. Children, you know, are often striking likenesses of their parents; and in their minds and habits, they likewise often resemble them. You should strive then to be good, not from mere self-love, and that you may get to heaven, but because your duty to others requires it.

Earl Granville, when laying the foundation stone of the Alexandria Orphanage, in England, thus expressed himself in reference to the great value of children:—'Few will deny that a child is "an inestimable loan," as it has been called, or refuse to acknowledge, with one of our greatest poets, that "the world would be somewhat a melancholy one if there were no children to gladen it." Children, more then any other earthly thing, equalise the conditions of society—to rich and poor they bring an interest, a pleasure, and an elevation, which nothing else that is earthly does.'

Now young people, before they think of engaging themselves, should clearly know each other's peculiar views of religion; because if they differ seriously on this point, there is danger of its interfering with that full confidence which is so essential to happiness.

CHAPTER XI.

SEXUAL INTERCOURSE—ITS LAWS AND CONDITIONS—ITS USE AND ABUSE.

There is an increasing and alarming prevalence of nervous ailments, and complicated disorders, that **could be** traced to **have** their sole origin from this source. Hypochondria, in its various phases, results **from the premature and unnatural waste of the** seminal **fluid.** There speedily ensues a lack of natural heat, a deficiency of vital power, and consequently indigestion, melancholy, languor, and dejection ensue, the victim becomes enervated and spiritless, loses the very attributes of man and premature old age soon follows.

It is a prevalent error, that it is necessary for the semen **to be** ejected at certain times from the body—that its retention is incompatible with sound health and vigor **of** body and mind. **This is** a very fallacious idea. The seminal fluid is too precious, Nature bestows too much care in its elaboration, for it to be wasted **in** this unproductive manner. It is intended, when not used for the purpose of procreation, to be re-absorbed again into the system, giving vigor of body, strength and elasticity to the mind, making the individual strong, active and self-reliant. When kept as Nature intended, it is a perpetual fountain of life and energy—a vital force which acts in every direction—a motive power, which infuses manhood into every organ of the brain and every fibre of the body.

The law **of sexual morality** for childhood is one of utter negation of sex. Every child **should be** kept pure and free from amative excitement, and the least **amative** indulgence, **which is** unnatural and doubly hurtful. **No language** is strong enough to express the evils of amative excitement and unnatural indulgence before the age of **puberty;** and the dangers are so great that I see no way so safe as thorough instruction regarding them at the earliest age. A child may be taught, simply as a matter of science, as one learns **botany, all that is** needful **to know, and** such knowledge may protect it from the **most terrible evils.**

The law for childhood is perfect purity, which cannot be too carefully guarded and protected by parents, teachers, and all care-takers. The law for youth is perfect continence—a pure vestalate alike in both sexes. No indulgence is required by one more than the other—for both Nature has made the same provision. The natures of both are alike, and any—the least—exercise of the amative function is an injury to one as to the other. Men expect that women shall come to them in marriage chaste and pure from the least defilement. Women have a right to expect the same of their husbands. Here the sexes are upon a perfect equality.

On this subject, Dr. Carpenter, in his physiological works, has written like a man of true science, and therefore of true morality. He lays it down as an axiom that *the development of the individual, and the reproduction of the species, stand in an inverse ratio to each other.* He says:—"The augmented development of the generative organs at puberty can only be rightly regarded as *preparatory* to the exercise of the organs. The development of the *individual* must be completed before the procreative power can properly be exercised for the continuance of the race." And in the following extract from his "Principles of Human Physiology,' he confirms my statement respecting the unscientific and libertine advice of too many physicians : " The author would say to those of his younger readers, who urge the wants of nature as an excuse for the illicit gratification of the sexual passions, ' Try the effects of *close mental application* to some of those ennobling pursuits to which your profession introduces you, in combination with *vigor-ous bodily exercise*, before you assert that appetite is unrestrain-able, and act upon that assertion.' Nothing tends so much to increase the desire as the continual direction of the mind toward the objects of its gratification, whilst nothing so effectually re-presses it as a determined exercise of the mental faculties upon other objects, and the expenditure of nervous energy in other channels. Some works which have issued from the medical press contain much that is calculated to excite, rather than to re-press, the propensity ; and the advice sometimes given by practi-tioners to their patients is immoral, as well as unscientific."

Every man and every woman, living simply, purely, and tem-perately—respecting the laws of health in regard to air, food, dress, exercise, and habits of life, not only can live in the continence of a pure virgin life when single, and in the chastity which should be observed by all married partners—but be stronger, happier, every way better by so living.

Chastity is the conservation of life and the consecration of its **forces** to the highest use. Sensuality is the waste **of life and the degradation of its forces to pleasure** divorced from use. **Chastity** is life—sensuality is death.

From the age of puberty to marriage the law is the same for both sexes. Full employment of mind and body, temperance, purity, and perfect chastity **in thought, word, and deed.** The law is one of perfect **equality. There is no license for the male** which is **not equally the right of the female. There is no physiological ground for any indulgence in one case more than in the other. No man has any more right** to require or expect purity **in the** woman **who** is to be **his wife, than** the woman has **to** require and expect purity in her husband. It is a simple matter of justice and right No man can enter upon an amative relation with a woman except in marriage, without manifest injustice to his future wife, unless he allow her the same liberty; **and also** without a great wrong to the woman, and to her possible husband.

It is contended that the **sins of** men against chastity are more **venial than those of women, because of the liability of** women to **have children. But men are also liable to be the fathers of** children ; **and they are deeply wronged by** the absence of paternal care. The child has its rights, and every child has the right **to be** born in honest, respectable wedlock, of parents able to give **it a sound** constitution and the nurture and education it requires. **The child who lacks these conditions is grievously wronged by both father and mother.**

The law of **marriage is, that** a mature man and woman, with sound health pure lives, **and a** reasonable prospect of comfortably educating a family, when drawn to each other by the attraction of a mutual love, should chastely and temperately unite for **offspring. 'The** sexual relation has this chief and **controlling purpose. The law of nature is intercourse for reproduction. Under** the Christian law, **marriage is the symbol of the union of** Christ **with the Church; husband and wife** are one in the Lord ; they are to live in marriage chastity, not in lust and uncleanness; and there cannot be a more hideous violation of Christian morals than for a husband to wreck his sensuality upon a feeble wife against her wishes, and when she has no desire for offspring, and no power to give them the healthy constitutions and maternal care which is their right.

The law of Christian morality is very **clear.** It is the sexual union first and chiefly for its principal object. It is for the husband to refrain from it whenever it is not desired; whenever it would be hurtful to either; whenever it would be a waste of life; whenever it would injure mother and child, as during pregnancy and lactation. A man who truly loves a woman, must respect and reverence her, and cannot make her the victim of his inordinate and unbridled, selfish and sensual nature. He will be ever, from the first moment of joyful possession, to the last of his life, tender, delicate, considerate, deferent, yielding to her slightest wishes in the domain of love, and never encroaching, never trespassing upon, never victimizing the wife of his bosom, and the mother of his babes. We have romance before marriage—we want more chivalry in marriage.

This is not the world's morality—yet it seems to me the world must respect it. This high and pure Christian morality is not always enforced by Christian ministers, some of whom yield too much to human sensuality and depravity, instead of maintaining the higher law of Christian purity—which is but nature restored, or freed from its stains of sin. The world requires that unmarried women should be chaste, while it gives almost unbridled license to men. A girl detected in amours is disgraced and often made an outcast. In young men such irregularities are freely tolerated. They are "a little wild;" they "sow their wild oats;" but open profligacy, the seduction of innocence, the ruin of poor girls, adultery, harlotry and its diseases do not hinder men from marrying, nor from requiring that those they marry should have spotless reputations. It is not for a moment permitted that women in these matters should behave like men; and a pure girl is given to the arms of a wasted debauchee, and her babes are perhaps born dead, or suffer through life with syphilitic diseases, while she endures a long martyrdom from disordered, diseased, and unrestrained sensuality. For the unmarried, young men, soldiers, sailors, and all who do not choose to bear the burdens of a family, society has its armies of prostitutes—women like others, and more

than others, or in less reputable fashion, the victims of the unbridled lusts of man. These are everywhere tolerated as, "necessary evils," and, in some places, protected or regulated, and from
economical or philanthropic considerations, or both, combined
efforts are made to free them from the contagious diseases, which
for some centuries have been a curse attending this form of the
violation of the laws of nature—one of the consequences of lust,
which is the divorce of the sexual instinct from its natural use
and purpose.

The Christian law of marriage, as set down in the Holy Scrip-
tures, and defined by the best writers on moral theology, is in
harmony with nature—in consonance with the higher nature of
man. " God hath set the earth in families." Adultery is a sin,
because it disorders that divine arrangement. Selfish lust is a
sin, because it mars it. Fornication is a sin, because it prevents
pure marriages. Prostitution is a sin, because it is a sacrifice of
women, who might be wives and mothers, to the selfish lusts of
men. All useless indulgence is a waste of life, and a kind of
suicide. In a pure marriage union men and women unite themselves with God in acts of creative power.

The progress of humanity depends upon individual development, and the conditions of generation and gestation. With culture, and a harmonized development, we acquire a higher and
more integral life. When two parents are in their highest condition, and in a true union with each other, the child combines the
best qualities of both parents. When parents are not in the
unity of a mutual love, the child may be inferior to either parent.
The intensity of mutual love tends to the reproduction of
the best faculties of both parents in the child. When men or
women are exhausted or diseased the race deteriorates. Health
is therefore one of the conditions of progress.

" It is all very fine," I shall be told, " to talk of purity and
chastity ; but we must take men as they are. How are you going
to make men pure and chaste, and respectful of the purity of
women ? " How can you get men with strong amative propensities to live like anchorites ? "

How can you get men to do any right thing or refrain from any
wrong thing ? There are three motives—fear of punishment,
hope of reward, and sense of right, or the principle of duty.

The first of these is the lowest, but often the most effectual ; the second is higher, and appeals to hope and the love of happiness ; the third, the highest of all motives, pure and unselfish as the love of truth, as in mathematics, acts on noble minds with great power. Men of real conscientiousness love the right for its own sake. They are just from love of justice—pure from a sense and love of purity. They love good, and God as the source of all good ; and do right, not from fear or hope, but from pure love.

We must appeal to all motives. Men refrain from theft and other dishonest conduct from the dread of disgrace and punishment ; because they see that "honesty is the best policy," and from a sense of justice and regard to the rights of property, or a sense of honor which makes a mean action impossible. By similar motives great numbers are restrained from drunkenness and other vices. Children are to be restrained from impurity by the fear of the terrible consequences of unnatural indulgence in causing disease and pain, by the hope of a pure, healthy, and happy life of love in manhood and womanhood, and by a sense of the beauty and holiness of chastity, and the sacredness of the functions by which the race is re-created and preserved. The religious feelings that our bodies are to be kept pure, healthy, and holy in every way as " the temples of the Holy Ghost," cannot be too early instilled into the infant mind, which is open to the highest sentiments of veneration, devotion, and heroic religion. In youth there are the same motives. Indulgence in solitary vice is self-destructive of all that youth most values—a profanation of his own body. Seduction is a desecration of what he should hold in the most tender reverence. To the young man womanhood should be sacred, and every woman, mother, sister, the beloved of the present or the future, should never be wronged by one thought of impurity. In this matter instinct goes with right. The inward voice supports the outer law of morality. Before men can become bad, their instinctive modesty must be broken down. Unless very badly born, with disordered amativeness hereditary from a diseased and lustful parentage, they must be perverted and corrupted before they can act immodestly and impurely.

Women are protected by a strong public sentiment around them. They have the dread of disgrace. For them to yield to their own affectionate desires, or the solicitations of a lover, is a fall, is ruin. They have the hope of a loving husband, a happy home, and the respect of society. And in women passion has commonly less force, and the sentiment of modesty and purity **more power.** Women are weak in yielding to solicitation, giving **everything for love ; but we see how protective of female virtue** are these motives to vast numbers.

Men can perfectly **restrain** the **sensual part of their** natures whenever and wherever **they have a strong motive to do so. A** child would be simply mad **who was not controlled by the presence of father,** mother, **and persons** he **respected or feared. Young men have no difficulty when they are in company of pure women. They are in no trouble where their lives are full of mental and muscular activity, and particularly if their habits of** eating simply **and temperately, of** refraining **from** heating and exciting stimu- **lants, and** sleeping in cool beds and fresh air are such as health requires. There needs but the strong will to live **purely in any** one, and at any age—the will that comes **from the high motives** of conscience and religion, or all **motives** combined. **A strong** sense of what is **just** and **right controls** even the motions of our **bodies and actions which seem to be** involuntary. A man who **has a vivid sense of the right and duty of refraining** from sensu- **ality, and preserving his own purity of mind and** body, and the **chastity of all women, will do so even in his** dreams. When the **will is right, all things are soon brought into** its subjection. **The mind controls the organization, and the life forces** are directed **into other channels. A strong** man, **full of life and love, can safely hold a virgin in his arms and respect her** virginity, **if he have but the motives and the will to do so. If** he be pure in his will, how can he commit impurity? If **a woman** be sacred in his eyes, how can he profane her? It **is** not that men have not the power of self-restraint, the power to do right—it is that they lack **the** motive. They have lost the sense of right; **they are even im-** pelled **to do wrong by** the pressure **of** opinion around them. Boys **and young men are** driven **into libertinage by the** ridicule of their companions. **Vice is considered manly. They seek sen-** suality in an evil emulation, as they learn **to** smoke, or game, or drink. And, later on, **vanity has often more to do with** excess **than the force of lust. Young men seduce girls that they may** boast of it. They keep mistresses because it is the fashion. They exhaust themselves, because they wish to give a high idea of their manly prowess. Even in marriage women are injured, and have their health destroyed, yielding weakly, or from a false sense of duty, to a husband, whose own motive is the desire to acquit himself manfully in what he considers his marital duties. Men and women are, in thousands of cases, wretched victims to what they imagine to be the wants or expectations of each other. A man, ignorant of the nature of woman, and the laws of the generative function, goes on in a process of miserable exhaustion to please his wife; she submits, sometimes in pain, often in disgust, weariness, and weakness, to what she dare not from love or fear refuse.

Men have to know what is right, and to will to be right. This will is omnipotent. God helps those who have the will, who have e en the desire to do right.

If the presence of those we fear or reverence, respect or love, restrain us from sin, and stimulate us to right action, faith in the existence and presence of God, and angels, and the spirits of the departed, must have a more powerful and pervading influence. No one who really believes in the existence of a Supreme Being: no one who is strongly impressed with the reality of a Spiritual life, can go on doing what he knows to be wrong. A religious faith is therefore the most powerful of all restraints from evil, and incitements to good.

CHAPTER XII.

THE PARENT'S INFLUENCE IN DETERMINING THE PHYSICAL AND MORAL STATUS OF HIS CHILDREN.

How universal is the desire to get married—it is the great end and aim of life. There may be no change, in every possible point of view, so necessary to be previously well considered as matrimony; but yet how paramount to all others in man's history is the incentive which leads us on. It is indeed a most fertile theme, and volumes have been dedicated to this subject alone.

Our consideration herein of the question relates less to its obligations than its expediency, inasmuch as the main property of these remarks applies more to the issue than the individuals immediately concerned.

In thus premising that our reference is to the future and not to the past, it is useless repining at what we have made ourselves, except it be to let those who succeed us know the anguish we suffer for our own misdeeds, and by our representations induce them to avoid the hidden rocks on which we have foundered.

In advocating the guardianship of health, the father is held responsible for his child, not only for what he has made him, but also for what he may make of him. In this large world, however, three-fourths have to shift for themselves;—this address, therefore, is expressly dedicated to such, in order that they may see what is due from themselves, and how to repair the neglect these pages may find them suffering from.

In tracing the sick or delicate health of a child, or a growing lad, or a young man, to parental origin, supposing the father or mother to be made sensible that such is the case—that to themselves alone, or chiefly, have they to attribute their child's affliction, how painful must be their reflections! A parent's love for a child is the more active and fervent in proportion to such disadvantages, and therefore the more to be deplored is the calamity. A mother's grief and a father's regret—what can be more poignant, on witnessing their sinking or expiring offspring, especially when they know that, on giving it life, they conveyed to it the seeds of its premature dissolution? With such a fact constantly before us, how it behooves those anticipating unions to ponder before they perpetuate their own misery, if not for their own sakes and sufferings, at least in mercy to those who are to issue from their loins. What else can be expected from a couple where the combined health of the two is not equal to the ordinary health of one perfect individual? And how rarely do we really find, especially in all interesting matches, but that the bride or bridegroom is in what is termed "delicate health." Hence, oftentimes, the popular notion, that a pale-faced woman, or a "lovesick looking" young man, have only to marry to get well, instead of getting well first and marrying afterwards. A certain class of individuals are ever ready to ridicule this train of reasoning; but if they unhappily

disregard its application, they will be sure to. find out, when **too**
late, the truth to fall at their own doors. Hence, if there be any
truth in the statement, that children inherit the constitutions as
well as the features and minds of their parents, the imperative
and urgent necessity of young persons contemplating marriage,
to look before they leap, not only **at the** *trousseau* **or the** wife's
dowry, **or** the husband's estate and means, **but at the** stability
of each other's health. It is true, **marriage is oftentimes a remedy**
for certain ills, but only those ills begotten by **a disregard of**
natures ordinances; for it is as much a law at a certain age that
parties should marry, as that fishes should swim or birds should
fly; but then marriage is only timely, when consistently carried
out with regard to age and condition. It is monstrous when particular deformities, or fatal, though lingering sickness, exist at an
espousal.

We have **talked of the children** inheriting disease and delicate
health from their parents : the following **facts are striking corro-**
borations of how much, and principally **in that way, children**
take after their fathers and mothers ; **how not only health, form**
and feature, **but intellect and genius, or** imbecility and viciousness may be propagated. **The fact has** been long observed and
known, **but only** recently practically elucidated, **and** that most
satisfactorily, by Mr. Alexander Walker. **This gentleman has**
written extensively on matters connected **with the subject, but the**
book, whence **his** views are taken, is entitled " Intermarriage."
That portion under immediate notice relates to **the** resemblance
of progeny to parents.

The idea that it is possible. by appropriate marriages to secure
a certain standard of beauty, statute and form, unfortunately
does not secure that notice it is worthy of, because people **rarely**
think of the possibility until courtship has commenced ; but **the**
evidence presently to be offered **must convince the most sceptical**
and selfish that it is **of** most certain accomplishment, and, fur-
thermore, that so attractive are the results, that the reflective will
take care not to surrender their affections merely to love at sight,
while it is quite possible to command that powerful feeling when
well, equally as when ill-directed.

All parents, writes Mr. Walker, communicate distinct points of
resemblance to their children, and the part which each parent

takes is modified by the **similarity or** dissimilarity betwixt the **father and** mother ; **for instance, in** unions between persons of the same variety, such as where a similarity in complexion, form, make, and temperament, exists, certain fixed resemblances ensue in the issue thereof. Again, when persons of different complexions **and different** temperaments marry, the issue partake of different *points* of resemblance. Lastly, when persons of **the** same family (breeding *in and in,* as it is termed,) marry, the **issue** assume new features; he therefore divides his investigations **of** resemblances **betwixt parents and children into three varieties** which are as follows :

FIRSTLY,—When persons of the *same variety* marry, but of *different* families.

SECONDLY,—Where persons of *opposite variety* marry, also of *different* families.

THIRDLY,—Where persons of the *same family* intermarry.

In the first arrangement, where persons of the same variety marry, one parent communicates the *Anterior series* of resemblances, and the other the *Posterior;* but either parent may impart either series.

The Anterior series consists of the *Forehead,* and bony parts of the face, as

The Orbits,	Jaws,
Cheek Bones,	Chin and Teeth,

as well as the shape of the organs of sense, and the *tone* of the voice, and likewise *the whole of the internal* nutritive system which signifies the contents of the trunk, such as the lungs, heart, and digestive organs, as well as the form of the trunk.

The *Posterior* series consists of the *Back-head,* the few more moveable parts of the face, and the locomotive system, as—

The external Ear,	**Lower** part of the Nose,
Under Lip,	Eyebrows,

and the external forms of the body in so **far as they** depend on the muscles, as well as the form of the limbs, **even to** the *fingers, toes, nails,* etc.

Mr. Walker assigns reasons why certain organizations should go together, namely, from their connexion; such as, for instance, he says, that portion of the brain which *regulates* the senses, corresponds with them, and consequently influences their organization internal and external, and, in like manner, that **portion influencing the motive powers, namely the back-head, influences the form of the limbs, and hence the resemblance to that parent** in those particulars **which imparts either series.**

Various corroborations are found in Mr. **Walker's book to prove** this assertion. It **has been observed that in a female with a short** and round face, chubby cheeks, and **a full forehead, but "contracted and fine in the nose and mouth," the trunk will be found** wide and capacious, and **the limbs tapering; whilst, on the** contrary, women with slender **oval faces and aquiline noses, have** spare and slender bodies.

With a view of determining the truth of the statement of either parent giving a particular series of resemblances of themselves to their offspring, Mr. Walker recommends the various parts of the head and face of a child, as detailed in the subjoined columns, to be examined, and those points not possessed by the child as resembling either father or mother to be crossed out, and those resembling to remain, when it will at once be seen which parent the child takes after, **and from which the** *anterior* or *posterior* series is derived.

NAMES OR INITIALS OF CHILD.

PARTS RESEMBLING THE MOTHER.	PARTS RESEMBLING THE FATHER.
Forehead.	Forehead.
Upper middle part of Head.	Upper middle part of head.
Bony parts of Face.	Bony parts of Face.
Teeth.	Teeth.
Digestive System.	Digestive System.
Form of Eyes. *Eyebrows.* *Middle of Nose. Point of Nose. Upper Lip. Under Lip.*	Form of Eyes. *Eyebrows.* *Middle of Nose. Point of Nose. Upper Lip. Under Lip.*
Ears. Back-head.	Ears. Back-head.
Upper middle part of Head, over the Ears, and towards the Temples.	Upper middle part of Head, over the Ears, and towards the Temples.
Frontal Protuberances.	Frontal Protuberances.
Chest. Limbs.	Chest. Limbs.
Fingers, Toes, Nails.	Fingers, Toes, Nails.

Those **parts printed** in italics are variable, **by the cerebral** (back part of brain so called) influencing the **muscles more or** less connected with them.

In examining resemblances, the *front face* of a child may resemble one parent, but the *profile* will resemble the other.

The *front view* best displays the observing faculties; the *profile view*, the *active* **ones.**

" The parent who gives the *locomotive* system, does not give the **carriage and the manner of walking.** These are always given by **the other** parent, who gives the organ of sense." Therefore the child with the limbs in resemblance of the mother walks like the father, and *vice versâ,* as the eye directs the walking, **and gives** the character to it. Witness **the step of** the countryman, or the man **of fashion.** " **The transmission of the mind is derived in equal and distinct portions from both parents, when parents are of the same variety, and the temper and disposition in like manner ; but one gives the whole of the nutrative, and the other the whole of the locomotive organs.**"

The child who resembles the anterior series of the one parent, is also characterized by a corresponding similarity in the functions of taste, smell, sight, etc., and also the observing, imitating, acquiring, and other faculties. The *back-head,* or posterior **series, im**parts the *passions* **and** *appetites.*

" **Whatever increases the** ardor of passion, invigorates the pro**geny "—this shows the indispensability of** health in **parties mar**rying. **The condition of health, the occupation, the state of mind, whether happy or saddened, at the period of matrimony, all have an influence upon the offspring. In the** excitement pres**ent, whether it be intellectual or sensual, whether** it be the **gentle emotion of pure affection, or the burning passion of mere desire, how necessarily must the consequences** fall upon the issue **thereof.**

How important, then, is it to select the most fitting period **of** life, when the **intellect is ripest, when the health** is most perfect, and when circumstances **combine to diffuse the greatest amount** of happiness to bride and bridegroom ; how important **is it to** select that period for marriage, and how equally important after **what has been** stated, **that the** *mind and health* **of** one parent, and **the** *appetites, passions and figure* **of** the other, **are perpetuated in** **the offspring, that the selection should** be a **judicious one, and made only with reflection and forethought ?**

We now come to speak of the second variety, called, in agricultural phraseology, "The Law of Crossing," which is where parties marry who are of different temperament and characters. In the former instance, it was stated, that where the father and mother were of the same variety, *either* parent might communicate **the** resemblances which went together, namely, *mind* and *health*—or the *forehead* and *digestive organs*, etc., and the *back-head*, or *will* or *appetites* and *form of limbs*, etc.

Now, where parties of different breeds marry, supposing them to be of equal age, vigor, etc., the MALE gives the *back-head* and *locomotive organs*, and the FEMALE gives the *face* and *nutritive organs*.

Hence, in "cross" alliances, the intellect of the mother, and the animal power of the father, descend usually to the offspring, except in especial cases, which are explicable on the principle, that power imparts power, and debility, debility.

The inference from this statement is, that in healthy alliances with persons of different variety, the father gives the energy and the mother the intellect.

This is as it should be, and as such a union always commands the like results (which marriage among the same variety do not, for there *either* parent, be it remembered, may give *either* mind or strength), it follows that cross-breeds secure a more vigorous and healthy progeny, and hence are to be preferred. There are sundry modifications observable, even in the resemblances thus given; but they do not upset the positive law, that the father (the amount of health being equal) gives the character of the frame, and the mother the organs of sense.

The last variety is where the parents are both of the same family where the propagation is termed " breeding in and in."

"The third Law operates where *both parents* are not only of the same *variety*, but of the *same family in its narrowest sense*, and where the *female* GIVES ALWAYS the *back-head* and *locomotive organs*, and the *male* the *face* and *nutritive organs*," precisely the reverse of what takes place in crossing.

Agriculturists, sportsmen, cattle-breeders, and all persons concerned in the rearing of animals, are well aware that in these kinds of unions the race degenerates; and our own species are not exempt from the same law. Every person can attest the fact, by observing among his friends where such unions are preserved, as cousins intermarrying, and other **near relations, the** evident fall-ing off **in the issue, if any rise at all.**

An **appendage as to these curious** facts, Mr. **Walker considers that the sex of the child is more** usually determined by that pa-**rent imparting the vital system, subject to some exceptions.** The **prolific power of either sex depends** upon their relative state **of health.**

Thus, then, we observe the children take after their parents in equal proportions. A child will resemble its father in the *back* part of the head, and in that **portion of the frame** influenced by it, as the form **and stature, whereas it will take after its** mother in the *front* part **of the head and the vital system, or in other words, the health and existence.** Of course these resemblances **are modified by the** relationship, as **stated,** existing betwixt the **mother and father,** whether they be of the same variety, **or of the same family, or** of entirely different characteristics. The mar-riages **between** parties of the same variety do not produce such decisive results as among those of opposite variety ; **and those** among the same family are the least **prolific and healthy of the** range.

Now, it must be remembered that the parents giving the *intellect* **and** *existence,* **or the** *energy* **and** *form,* convey to their offspring **the peculiarities of their own organization.** The power of repro-**ducing the species accompanies the vital system, and only** in pro-**portion to the perfection** of the latter is the perfection of the **former ; hence, if a** parent, **in** infirm health, with peculiar ner-**vous or** other derangements, happen to perpetuate **in his own child the** *anterior series*—namely, *intellect* and the nutritive system, what **can be** expected **in the ensuing** generation, should that child sur-vive, or in **his turn marry or** become a parent ? The same result would follow, and the degeneracy **at last** would end in the cessa-tion of further extension, and **the** race of such would become extinct. To those who perfectly understand these remarks and their application, many circumstances connected with their own health become immediately **explicable, which** before **were matters of wonderment, how** such **and such could be.** The inference shows how dependent **the negative system of man is upon the** general health, and **how much that rests upon** ancestral origin.

CHAPTER XIII.

DOMESTIC INFELICITY—ITS CAUSE AND ITS CURE.

Matrimony is a condition congenial with our nature. It is a main incident in human happiness. Even the birds pair, and what a reproof that should be to all obstinate bachelors and old maids. Apart from the feelings which generate love, and which make men go through fire and water to obtain the object of their affection, and which urge women to leave happy and wealthy homes to realize their sympathy and devotion, there is a great feeling in the circumstance of the mere communion—in the social friendship betwixt man and wife, which can exist nowhere else in like degree; apart from the ties of offspring that may bless a union, the fact of the worldly partnership, and the necessary mutual confidence existing in all matters of domestic and political economy, cement the compact, and render marriage the fastest attachment in the world. Hence the delightful position, above all price, of a pair well and suitably allied to each other in marriage. Much is necessary to be known with a view to discriminate between evil and good; to foretell happiness or misery. How different are men's feelings upon the subject at twenty and thirty. There is no trial beforehand of character and disposition. Marriage is a hit or miss; the shot when once fired cannot be recalled. Courtship is a very artificial criterion; the face is lighted up with its best smiles and wears its cleanest aspect—every flaw is concealed—not a stray curl is suffered to hang out of place—the voice assumes its most melodious tones—the very gait is graceful—the picture is handsomely framed—and the conquest is complete. Both sexes adopt the like manoeuvre, and both frequently disappoint each other.

"*Men are April when they woo*—December when they wed. Maids are May when they are maids, but the sky changes when they are wives.*"

Young people usually pride themselves upon being the best judges of what and who is most suitable. Courtship is an affair that advice is seldom sought in, and, should it be tendered, is rarely acceptable; it is hard to counsel upon, but the prudent will at least reflect, lest they be too precipitate, and should not disregard the counsel that persons authorized may tender. It is somewhat curious that all imaginative writers, such as romance manufacturers and novel concocters, represent fathers as obdurate and hard-hearted, and mothers as inimical generally to their children's choice. The notion is a false one and ill-timed; for who can feel such interest, such dear solicitude for their children's prosperity and happiness as the authors of their being?

What a void in an old man's heart is a disobedient and ungrateful child! How hard it is to regulate these matters! Young folks do not for a moment recollect that their parents may have been lovers, and must have acquired some experience worth detailing. Certainly, an immensity depends on a good example being set at home—care in excluding unsuitable acquaintances for our children, and caution and yet an interest in introducing others.

But the subject I have entered upon is where the noose is tied, whence there is no escape—whence all hope of a change, except that brought about by mutual or principal forbearance, is absent; I allude to domestic infelicity. Of course, there are a thousand and possible more provocatives to family jars and dissensions that render a married life a most formidable, and continuous warfare.

What is the principal and provoking cause to marital infelicity —to perpetual squabbles—to family discomfort—to neglect of home—let us add, to ruin, desolation and beggary? We shall not be far wrong in attributing the majority to two especial common and prevalent vices, namely, drunkenness and irascibility of temper. In dividing them, in justice we must lay the blame of the former principally to the husband, the latter to the wife. Of course the tables are sometimes turned, and there are exceptions to both conditions. To these two evils I purpose confining my remarks and suggestions for their alterations, if not for their removal.

A man may take to drinking through want of comfort at home, and the woman may acquire a bad temper through a husband's neglect; it is impossible to go into the very many inquiries of the why, and how, and what is the cause; else we must canvass over personal dislikes, jealousies, opposing habits, physical inaptitudes, disparity of ages, family interpositions, &c. We come to this fact; hundreds and hundreds of men are drunkards, and thousands of women are plagued with terrible irascible dispositions. What is the remedy?

The companion to a drunken mate is the worst off, because the drunkard sooner falls into that state of health that the stimulus comes to be his only support, and his physical condition is a hell to him without his soul-spoiling antidote ; reason and reflection are of little use to a depraved habit. The consequences are the more likely to bring him to his senses, and these consequences are general bodily suffering, extreme ill-health, and loss of business. It is well, where friends and relations will interpose and express their indignation and show their displeasure, and perhaps well-expressed contempt may create a thought at least towards reformation. Coercion, if the nearest of kin might use it would no doubt have great influence. Drunkenness had best be punished by positive imprisonment, and why not? Offences less injurious to public morals are, and what is the object, but to prevent their repetition? Thanks. however, to the spirit of the age, inebriation is on the decline. It exists chiefly among the very ignorant and the badly brought up.

Now let us just view the consequences of irascibility of temper. I need not picture the dreariness or the constant confusion of a home beset with continued quarrels. That such things are, every day tells of them. If we read them not in the public journals, we learn of them through the travel of small talk—through scandal and other channels, and many of us know more or less from nearer sources the truth of such a report.

In irascibility of temper, there are two things to be considered. By no means to aggravate it, and by all means to try and subdue it. In whomsoever the fault rests, the other should not fan the flame. Suppose we throw the blame on the weaker of the two sexes ; the only alternative is to treat it with forbearance. A despairing man will dole out his lamentations to the effect that he is the most wretched of all living creatures—that he has no peace —that the maxim so often broached is reversed, and whatever is, is wrong—"that his wife has the most turbulent, restless, dissatisfied, worst temper in the world"—that she either sulks or raves —that no cat and dog were ever such bitter antagonists as his spouse and himself ; his very detail provokes a smile, but alas, it is too true, and his position is indeed a most miserable one. An indignant man will exclaim—*he* would not put up with it : *he* would soon show who was master. Such a feeling, such a disposition, and such a mode of proceeding is rarely successful. In the struggle for mastership hard words lead to fistycuffs, tearing of caps, and abusive language—language bad to use, and worse to utter before children. As well attempt to quench fire with oil, or carry water in a sieve, as to subdue the temper of a willful woman by hard means, such as by her own weapon—an unruly tongue. Irascibility is temporary insanity. And a woman when thus wild and ungovernable is unquestionably mad. And how altered now is the treatment of the insane; straitjackets, belts, iron bands, hand-cuffs, and wooden stocks, are supplanted by mild physical restraint, gentle persuasion, and every possible show of kindness. It will do the heart good to learn that humanity and benevolence and generous forbearance, with coaxing and solicitation firmly exercised, have entirely superseded the lash, the threat, and (one can happily add) the torture of by-gone times. "Have a wife and rule a wife" makes a good comedy where the parts are set down, but the acting is not modelled in nature. No wife should take advantage of this advice and refer to these hints to husbands as sanctioning her viciousness of disposition, for the remarks may apply to herself, and be as practically in request by her companion ; but the benedict may rely upon it that forbearance is his best shield of defence: the attacks rebound from it. An angry and contentious woman will have the last word, and so long as the husband provokes the argument, so long will it be kept up. Never mind the sharp hits of a wife's malice; so long as you know you do not deserve them, you can afford to bear them, and if you know you merit them, you had best be silent. If you know such and such a theme is a tender point, never broach it. If you are well aware that keeping the dinner waiting, staying out past your time, introducing smoking in your parlor, having noisy friends who provoke you to stay up late, giving bachelor parties, offend and bring upon you all the domestic uneasiness possible, all I can say is, you are very foolish to do these things, and after all, you can easily abandon such practices without much detriment to yourself. If your mind be the stronger of the two, and you value peace and quietness at home, cultivate pursuits more pleasing to your wife, and you will most likely ensure your object ; this kind of forbearance will be certain to succeed in the long run. Husbands cannot expect to have everything their own way ; they must give and take; they may talk of their supremacy, their being the prop of the house, the support of the family— and they will lived to be asked by the wife, who else should be? So it goes for nothing, and the man had best hold his tongue.

No, my friend, if you are a melancholy, and hypochondriacal, and yet disputatious man, and have a disputatious spitfire of a wife, I do not envy you your position; but of this I am sure, and I have *seen* a great deal of it although I do not confess to be a party in the drama, that *kindness, concession,* and *quiet reasoning,* and, if that won't do, *generous forbearance* is the only loophole of escape you have. If, madam—supposing my reader a lady—the remarks apply to yourself, as the self-willed or the abused, pray interpret good naturedly my suggestions. I am an advocate for a woman's rights, and I contend that a husband should be respected. I abhor oppression and cruelty, and would recommend no one tamely to submit to be trampled upon, but I know the virtue of concession, and the value of mutual forgiveness. Most irascible people are otherwise amiable and benevolent.

In Montgomery's "Law of Kindness" is given an anecdote of an irascible man denying himself to a Quaker, whom he at the same time abused by the epithet of "rascal," bidding him begone. The Quaker mildly replied, " *Well, my friend,* may God put thee in a *better* mind." The angry man was subdued by the kindness of the reply, and, after a careful consideration, became convinced he was wrong. He sent for the Quaker, and after making a humble apology, he said, "How were you able to bear my abuse with so much patience?" "Friend," replied the Quaker, " *I will tell thee. I was naturally as violent and hot* as thou *art; but I knew that to indulge my temper was sinful,* and also *very foolish.* I observed that *men in a passion* always spoke very *loud, and I thought if I could control my voice,* I should keep down my passion. *I therefore made a rule never to let* it rise above a certain key; and, by a *careful observance of this rule,* I have, *with the blessing of God, entirely mastered my natural temper.*

We may depend upon it, kindness is the best rod. The Christian motto is—

"Overcome evil with good."

If properly carried out, it is a key which opens the hearts of all around us, giving us a place in their affections. It will disarm anger of its power, hatred of its sting, enmity of its opposition, and sarcasm of its malice; *it will make the communion of husband and wife* more tender; it will secure the obedience of children; it will make the ties of friendship strong; it will turn enmity into benevolent feeling; it will minister to the widow and the orphan, in the pitiless storms of winter; and it will look to the comfort of the dumb beasts who serve us, saving them from cruelty, and ensuring them good treatment. All this it will do if practiced; and if not the nearest road, it is the easiest way, to be Happy.

Lastly, if forbearance, if kindness, if, indeed, continued submission secure you not tranquility, resort at once to separation. If you cannot effect it by mutual consent, call in the aid of your nearest friends, and carry it out peremptorily. Let there be no truce; when once you resolve upon it, *do it.* A miserable home is bad for the wife, shocking for the family, and deplorable for the husband. By separation, surely, all the contention, and sparring, and jarring is at an end, and then our several philosophy must be to rest content; for, terrible as the isolation to a domestic party may be, it is much better than to be in perpetual war.

Thus far I have principally contended for the wife; thus far I have advised the husband to forego his authority and privileges; thus far I have contended for submission from the stronger to the weaker vessel, so that the lady cannot object to receive a parting word of advice to herself. Let every wife whose husband loves other places than his own home, or rather what should be his home, examine how far she imitates Peggy or Jenny. Jenny is all scepticism, and scarcely believes men can be honest; she doubts their fidelity, distrusts their steadiness of purpose, and anticipates nought but beggary and want.

> "O, heaven! were man
> But constant, he were perfect; that one error
> Fills him with faults."

Such she believed awaited her choice, and thus she bid

"Dear Meg, be wise, and live a single life,
Troth, it's nae mows to be a married wife."

Peggy draws a livelier **picture** of the married state. She believes
a husband may be **won to constancy** ; she thinks, if *he* errs,

"*It's ten to ane the wives are maist to blame.*"

She places great faith in

"*A bleezing ingle and a clean hearth stane.*"

And, last of all, she exclaims, inclusive of her best efforts to attract and please—

"*Good humour and while begonets shall be
Guards to my face to keep his love for me.*"

And **doubtlessly** these are sinister contrivances to win a man's
heart. The idea at once brings to the mind the delights of **our**
"ain fireside."

"Blest winter nights ! **when, as the genial fire**
Cheers the wide hall, **our cordial family**
With soft domestic arts the hours beguile."

The disposition would impel me, in the pleasing thoughts of such
a scene, to disbelieve a woman wanting in her contribution to so
much comfort ; but we gather knowledge as we **move along, and**
facts are too numerous to leave a doubt about it. Katherine (the
subdued wife of Pertruchio) thus breaths her recantation, and
advises one of her own sex in the following strain. It expresses
all that can be said on such an occasion, and husbands might club
together to **have a series of cards** printed with the admonition
thereon, for presentation to unruly wives :

THE WIFE'S DUTY TO HER HUSBAND.

"Fie, fie ! unknit that threatening unkind bow ;
And dart not scornful glances from those eyes,
To wound thy lord, thy king, thy governor;
It blots thy beauty, as frosts bite the meads;
Confounds thy fame, as whirlwinds shake fair buds;
And in no sense is meek or amiable.
A woman moved is like a fountain troubled,
Muddy, ill-seeming, thick, bereft of beauty;

And while it is so, none so dry or thirsty
Will design to sip, or touch one drop of it.
Thy husband is thy lord, thy life, thy keeper,
Thy head,.thy sovereign; one that cares for thee
And for thy maintenance, commits his body
To painful labor both by sea and land;
To watch the night in storms, the day in cold,
While thou liest warm at home, secure and safe
And craves no other tribute at thy hands.
But love, fair looks, and true obedience;—
Too little payment for so great a debt.
Such duty as the subject owes the prince,
Even such a woman oweth to her husband;
And when she's froward, peevish, sullen, sour,
And not obedient to his honest will,
What is she but a foul, contending rebel,
And graceless traitor to her loving lord?—
I am ashamed that women are so simple
To offer war where they should kneel for peace!
Or seek for rule, supremacy, and sway,
When they are bound to serve, love, and obey."

CHAPTER XIV.

VENEREAL OR SEXUAL DISEASES.

Of the multitude of diseases which the human frame is liable
to, none cause so much misery, moral and physical, as those
called venereal. Many a thoughtless youth has in a moment of
temptation given way to his passions and thus filled his system
with corruption, which may never leave him to the end of his life,
or what is far worse, he has poisoned the fountain of his life, he
will leave it as a heritage of misery to his offspring or will taint
the blood of the partner of his bosom making her the innocent par-
taker of his disease. How many such are there in every locality,
dragging out a wretched existence, a misery to themselves and an
eyesore to society. They are left, as it were, by the Almighty to

warn others against vicious practices and point the moral of the
preacher against vice and immorality.

GONORRHŒA OR **CLAP.**

This is an inflammation of the mucous membrane of the sexual
organs, accompanied by a discharge, the result of impure connection.

The symptoms of clap are as follows: shortly after the infection
has been communicated, usually from three to eight days, a sensation of heat and uneasiness is experienced in the end of the
penis, accompanied generally with a little redness and difficulty in
passing water, in a day or two the discharge of matter increases,
and becomes thinner and of a greenish or yellowish color, sometimes tinged with blood.

The head of the penis is red and inflamed, and the urine occasions a scalding pain. When the inflammation extends to the
bladder, there is a distressing desire to pass water, with a constant
uneasiness about the testicles, and between the legs. When the
inflammation is high it produces what is called chordee, in which
the penis is in a state of erection, and is curved downward with
great pain; this occurs generally when the patient is warm in
bed.

From the inflammation, phimosis may ensue, in which the
foreskin is hard and swollen so that it cannot be drawn back;
or, when the swelling takes place behind the head it cannot be
drawn forward and is called paraphimosis.

The glands of the groin sometimes swell and inflame, as well
as the testicles.

Gleet is the result of gonorrhœa, and proceeds into the chronic
form, after active inflammation has subsided. It is sometimes
very obstinate. Another result of gonorrhœa is stricture, which
is a partial closing up of the urethra, or passage leading from
the bladder; this may be known by the stream of water becoming
flattened or twisted, like a gimlet, or forked.

Stricture causes much pain and inconvenience, and often, if
not promptly cured, troubles the sufferer at various times during
his whole life.

If the discharge be suffered to remain on the glans of the
penis, or on the outside of the foreskin, excoriations, chaps and
warts spring up speedily and plentifully, and protrude before the
prepuce, or sometimes become adherent to it; it therefore shows
how necessary cleanliness is in these disagreeable complaints, to
escape the vexations alluded to. The earliest symptoms should
always be attended to, and where there is the least suspicion that
the disease has been contracted, (and all indulgence outside of
wedlock is fraught with the greatest danger and risk), prompt
and energetic action must be taken.

It is of the first importance to nip, if possible, the disease in its
bud; and that this can be done frequently and successfully the
adoption of the following method will prove.

TREATMENT.

Immediately on the advent of the first symptoms, or as soon as
there is reason to believe that the party must have received the
infection, throw up an injection of the nitrate of silver.
Take of nitrate of silver, 1 scruple; distilled water 1 ounce,
mix, and strain through blotting paper. Pour a small quantity
of the solution into a wine-glass; procure a small glass syringe,
fill the same with the preparation; carefully insert the point
of the syringe into the urethra, and allowing the penis
to rest loosely, press the piston of the syringe, and inject the
contents. Hold the syringe still for half a minute, to retain the
solution in the urethra, and then suffer it to escape. There is
generally some difficulty to a patient's applying an injection for
the first time, and there is usually an apprehension lest he force
the injection into the bladder—there is little fear of that occur-
ing, first owing to the general awkwardness, and secondly, to the
natural resistance which the introduction of a stimulating fluid to
a sensitive and resistive passage meets with. If the least pain or
sense of distension ensue, the best plan is to withdraw the syringe,
supposing half of the injection only to have been thrown up, and
suffer the injected fluid to return, and then to apply the remainder. The disease being rarely seated beyond a couple of inches
at the onset, there is no need of the injection higher up, but the
use of the injections generally, as it is just possible that an in-

jection might enter the bladder and it might not be advisable that
it should go there, the pressure of the finger against the *Perineum*,
during the operation, will prevent any fluid passing that spot.
The introduction of a syringe, if carefully resorted to, seldom
gives any pain—the orifice of the urethra is of course tender, and
no violence should be used, and it is as well to dip, previously,
the point of the syringe in a little sweet oil. On the withdrawal
of the syringe and escape of the injection, a slight burning sensation is experienced, which soon subsides, and no further inconvenience is occasioned, until called upon to urinate, when a smart
scalding is felt, and the last few drops of the urine may bring a
spot or two of blood. Succeeding to or before the act of micturition, if it be long deferred, there occurs rather a copious
yellow discharge, which is given off from the membrane of the
urinary passage in consequence of the injection, and is not to be
considered as Gonorrhœal matter. This may be continued more
or less for some hours, but it generally subsides into a thin watery
secretion. The pain in passing water also goes off, and by night
time or the following morning the effects of the injection have
subsided. If the operation of the injection be ineffectual, the
Gonorrhœal discharge will, in all probability, rapidly succeed,
and with it the usual sensations of scalding and pain. It may
happen to the contrary—the Gonorrhœal symptoms may not have
advanced, and there may still remain the red and tender orifice
with a slight weeping. It is then prudent to repeat the injection,
which will be accompanied by the like result as before, but possibly less acute. Supposing the symptoms of Clap not to advance
and yet not wholly to subside, the operation may be repeated
once more. If, despite this third trial, much irritation ensue,
with great heat on urinating, or itching after it, and it be attended
with pain about the perineum, groin, or loins, or testicles, or no
amendment be perceptible, the injection had better not be
repeated, and the next and best step is immediately to relieve the
bowels by a full dose (1 ounce) of castor oil, and to follow the
action of the medicine by immersion in a warm bath, availing
also of frequent local hot fomentations, and then to treat the
disease in the ordinary way.

If, happily, as it very frequently does, the injection annihilate
the complaint—a warm bath or two—a day or two's quiet, with

temperate living (local support, by means of a suspensory bandage), and the avoidance of all stimuli, will find the patient perfectly convalescent.

If this treatment does not stop the disease, recourse must be had to other means to be used promptly.

A warm bath should be taken every second or third day. A suspensory bandage should be worn, the bowels kept open with castor oil and rest of body and mind strictly enjoined.

The common drink should be of the mildest diluents. Barley water and flax seed tea are the best drinks. Gruel is the next best repast ; it will do for the evening, and makes an excellent supper. Indeed, in very severe instances, gruel is the only nourishment that should be taken for several days.

Drinks should be of the simplest kind, such as will pass the more readily through the kidneys, and produce the mildest urine; hence, next to water, have we milk and water, weak tea, barley water, flax seed tea, gum water or gum arabic (the best quality) may be suffered to dissolve in the mouth, not exceeding an ounce or two in the day, for it is not very digestible, but with the common drinks swallowed from time to time, it unites, and possibly renders the urine less acrid. The various light soups are permissible such as vermicelli, macaroni, tapioca, and gruel broth. Sweets, pastries, solid dumplings, plum-puddings, cakes, and all those sorts of things are bad. The bread should be taken toasted and eaten cold ; or it may be sopped in warm tea, or warm milk. Porridge is not objectionable. The best bread, also, is the unfermented; and then, again, the "brown" is preferable to the "white." It helps to keep the bowels open, acts favorably on the kidneys, and at the same time, is very nourishing and palatable. Rusks, brown bread, biscuits and all the light farinaceous preparations are good. All salted meats, savory dishes, little surprises of delicacies, and "tit bits" must be avoided. The next and best help is bodily rest.

If a man could lay up for a week, it would nearly cure him. That, in ninety-nine cases out of a hundred, is impossible.

SCALDING.—Keep the bowels open with castor oil, and take the following sedative mixture.

Mucilaginous and Sedative Mixture.

Take of Bicarbonate of Potass, 1 **drachm** ; Mucilage of Acacia, 3 ounces ; Spirits of Sweet Nitre, 2 drachms ; **Tincture of** Henbane, 3 drachms; Syrup of Tolu, 3 drachms ; Distilled **water, 4 ounces.**

Mix.—Take three table-spoonsful **three times daily, morning,** noon, and night.

Purgation always relieves the scalding. Bathing the penis in warm water, as warm as it can well be borne, will ease the smarting in passing **urine** ; and if that fail, cold water may be found more effectual. Throwing up, must before urinating, a syringeful of a sedative injection, will help to allay the pain.

Sedative Injection to allay the Scalding and Pain.

Take of Extract of Belladonna, 10 grains ; Plain or Rose-water, 12 ounces. *Mix.*—Throw up **a** syringeful frequently in the day.

SURFACIAL DISCHARGE, AND ULCERATION **ONLY OF THE GLANS, PREPUCE, ETC.**

Where the discharge is traceable only to the Glans or Prepuce, and is or is not accompanied by cuticular excoriation, the application of a solution of the Nitrate of Silver will, in one or two "brushings," put a stop to the secretions, and the 'abrasive' invasion.

Solution of Nitrate of Silver.

Take of Nitrate of Silver ½ drachm ; **Distilled Water, 1** ounce. *Mix* **and** strain through blotting paper.—To be used with the feather end **of a pen.**

———

Solution of Sulphate of Zinc.

Take of Sulphate of Zinc, 1 scruple ; Pure Water, 1 pint. *Mix.*—Throw up between the nut and foreskin a syringeful of this application two or three times daily.

———

To return to the treatment of the discharge. As soon, however, as the scalding is on the wane, then may be taken the various preparations of Copaiba, Cubebs, and other particular remedies, which now, for the benefit of the patient, a series of prescriptions are offered, the headings of which will guide to their selection.

The ordinary Capsules of Copaiba.

Three may be taken three times daily—to be swallowed as boluses ; some people cannot take pills, but by merely half filling the mouth with water, and then throwing in what is to be swallowed, one "gulp" will take the whole down. This form of Copaiba spares the palate from the nauseous flavor of the medicine.

Cubebs.

Cubebs have been held as, and oftentimes they are, useful in Gonorrhœa. From two to three drachms of the Powder of Cubebs may be taken three times daily in water, observing the adjuncts of occasional purgatives, bland drinks, baths, and rest. If, however Cubebs do not produce a marked good in three or four days, it is useless continuing them.

Cubebs and Copaiba are both stimulants and diuretics, and, as far as we know, act on the mucous membranes ; but if carried beyond a certain effect, they irritate the kidneys, and produce considerable derangement. The following are severally good formulæ.

Copaibic and Cubebic Mixture.

Take of Balsam Copaiba, 1 ounce ; Mucilage of Acacia, 3 ounces ; Powder of Cubebs, ½ ounce; Spirits of Sweet Nitre, 2 drachms; Paregoric, 2 drachms; Simple Syrup, ½ ounce; Peppermint water sufficient to form a half pint mixture. Take two table-spoonsful twice or thrice daily.

Compound Copaibic Mixture.

Take of Honey, 1 ounce; Balsam Copaiba, 1 ounce; Powder of Acacia, 1 ounce; Liquor of Potass, 1 drachm; Mix, and add a little water gradually. Then, take of Tincture of Buchu, 1 ounce; Tincture of Cubebs, 1 ounce; Tincture of Opium, 30 drops. Peppermint or Cinnamon water sufficient to form a half-pint mixture. Take one or two table-spoonsful in a little water, two or three times daily. These are two excellent mixtures,

---

The Balsam Copaiba.

May be taken in doses of a tea-spoonful simply floated on water, or may be taken in half a glass of sherry. It may be made with magnesia into pills, and then ten to thirty swallowed in the day.

Preparation of Copaiba.

Copaiba is often prepared in the form of tincture and various other solutions (in an alkaline form among the rest), all of which are severally good; it is at best a nauseous preparation, and if it disagree, is apt to throw out over the body a species of nettle-rash, that is very irritable, and often alarming to a patient, who considers it to be a fearful advance of the disease—a suspension of the medicine, a dose of physic, and a warm bath or two, will completely put a stop to it. The copaiba must be recurred to very cautiously, or suspended entirely in case of a relapse.

PAIN AND DIFFICULTY IN PASSING URINE, WITH IRRITABILITY OF THE BLADDER, ETC., AND FREQUENT DESIRE TO URINATE.

These are the natural consequences of extended inflammation. They often occur from other causes than Clap; but with it they are rarely entirely absent.

These maladies are often aggravated as the discharge diminishes, or rather, the severer they are, the discharge becomes more or less suspended. Nature seldom allowing **two diseases** to proceed with equal virulence at the same time. The remediatory measures are principally sedatives, demulcents, baths, and rest. **Where** a **hardness or a tumor of the Perineum is present, leeches, warm fomentations, bran and** other poultices **are indispensable.** Cupping is an expedious and cleanly mode of relief in the earlier stages of severe pain thereabout.

In painful Micturition and frequent desire **of Urinate.**

Take of Camphor Julep, 8 ounces, Laudanum, 30 drops. *Mix.*—Take three table-spoonsful three times daily.

Demulcent Drink to facilitate the **Flow** *of Urine.*

Take of Barley-water, 2 pints; Nitrate of Potass. **2** scruples; **White** Sugar, 2 or three lumps. *Mix.*—Take a wine-glassful three **or four** times daily.

If the case resist the means recommended, and symptoms increase, medical aid *must be called in.*.

INFLAMMATION OF THE BLADDER.—PROSTRATE GLAND.— DISORDERED URINE.

This is so far beyond the control of a non-medical invalid, that it is scarcely prudent to allude to it; but the symptoms may be told **to** urge the employment of the professional man.

Inflammation of the mucous **lining of the bladder is** marked by the whey-looking appearance **of the** urine—pain **in** urinating; frequent desire to empty the **bladder; pain** about the situation **of** it, and considerable fever. The *Prostrate Gland* and neck of **the** bladder **become involved frequently** in the disturbance, and present **similar accompaniments, with** the **addition of great** suffering **in the perineum and rectum, a most pressing desire to void** water, **and yet inability to eject** more than a **drop or two at a time. Leeches, bleeding, and general active treatment, are in immediate requisition in such cases.**

CHORDEE.

This is a most painful affection, and is only present when the penis is distended or erect. When bleeding occurs, which it frequently does, it arises from some little vessel in the urinary passage giving way. The speediest way of deriving relief is by immersing the penis in cold water—or wrapping linen rags, dipped in the same, around the virile member. The pain is so intense, and the erection so constant when warm in bed, and the parts so very irritable, that the patient cannot sleep, and therefore it is advisable to administer sleeping draught and also to dip some lint in the embrocation and apply it to the under surface of the penis, going to bed with it on.

Sleeping Draught.

Take of Solution of Acetate of Ammonia, ½ ounce; Camphor Julep, 1 ounce; Spirits of Sweet Nitre, ½ drachm ; Tincture of Henbane, 1 drachm. *Mix.*—To form a draught to be taken at bed-time.

The Embrocation.—Poison.

Take of Opodeldoc, ½ ounce; Laudanum, ½ ounce. *Mix.*—Label it POISON and use it as advised—taking care it be not swallowed by mistake for the draught.

In obstinate cases of Chordee, leeches applied over the part will do good. The warm bath before going to bed will sometimes keep off the local excitement, and thereby allow sleep.

A pill composed of Camphor, 5 grains, and Belladonna, ½ grain, taken at bed time is highly beneficial.

Chordee will continue some time, and very much harass the individual, inducing frequently nocturnal emissions. Patience and persistence in the means suggested are the best antidotes.

SWELLING OF PREPUCE—PHYMOSIS.

A mere temporary enlargement is of no moment, although it shall attain treble or four times its ordinary bulk. In this instance, the Prepuce assumes a dropsical appearance, like a thin bladder filled with water, and is occasioned by what medical men call extravasated serum being deposited in the reticular membrane.

The treatment consists in the constant application of cold water, by means of lint moistened therewith and applied thereon— taking care to keep the penis well supported, rather than pendant. Syringing between the *Prepuce* and *Glans* with luke-warm water, milk and water, will help to subdue the inflammation. The swelling mostly subsides after a little while; where ulcerations exist on the glans, or warts, and are progressing, and fear is entertained lest a permanent adhesion between the foreskin and nut shall take place, then division, as the lesser of two evils, is necessary.

BUBO.

Buboes occur in Gonorrhœa, especially where there is any external irritation or excoriation around the glans. They consist of a slight swelling of the glans in the groin, but they really lead to abscesses, and consequently they are termed Sympathetic—they subside usually with the provoking cause. Warm fomentations, warm baths, and mild opening medicine are all that are required.

SWELLED TESTICLES.

Diseases of the testicles are so fraught with after-mischief, that the most prompt and skillful attention should be sought after. Immediately on discovery of a swelled testicle, the first step should be to procure a suspender—it gives instantaneous relief. The warm bath is also invaluable, and indispensable, and may be resorted to daily.

The next and speediest way of relieving swelled testicle is by bleeding from the arm or cupping in the loins, observing the strictest rest and abstinence. Some physicians advise emetics— all recommend purgatives; and saline aperients are most effectual. If bleeding and cupping be dispensed with, leeches can scarcely be withheld—but it is useless to apply them, except in large numbers. Frequent warm fomentations give great relief. The diet must be spare during this process, avoiding all wines, beer, and spirits. Let the patient secure as much bed-rest as possible. Let him also ride rather than walk when he can, and sit rather than stand. About the second or third day, when the inflammation shall have reached its height, still observing the same precautions. Use the Absorbent Mixture and keep up the secretion of the bowels. The testicles, or rather the scrotum, may be smeared or washed over, by means of a camel-hair brush, with the Tincture of Iodine (procure an ounce in a stopper vial) ; the operation will occasion some smarting, but it is only of very short duration. The application must be repeated night and morning, until the skin expoliates, or becomes too painful to be borne. As soon as the surface admits of its re-application, it must be renewed until the swelling disappears.

Absorbent Mixture.

Take of Iodide of Potass, ½ drachm; Distilled water, 7½ ounces; Tincture of Henbane, 2 drachms; Simple Syrup, 2 drachms. *Mix.*—Take three table-spoonsful three times daily. Each fresh bottle of mixture **may** have 10 **grains** extra **of the Iodide** of **Potass.**

GLEET.

Gonorrhœa proceeds from sexual intercourse and is infectious; but it may arise from a variety of other causes, drinking, sexual excesses, whether with females or from masturbation, accident, **or** ill-health; *Gleet is a subdued inflammation of the same kind, possessing more or less all the properties of the former,* although not so de-**terminately** infectious. Is Gleet curable? Unquestionably it **is** but by no specific Balsam, Elixir, or especial Simple. It must be treated with reference to the existing symptoms. It has to be re-peated and told, that the drainage is kept up by local irritation, by a loss of tone in the secreting vessels, by such a thing as sym-pathy with some neighboring or remote infirmity. This local ir-**ritation** may be removed by local application. There is a time when **the** mildest injections are promptly successful, whilst at others a cure only awaits the use of very active ones.

The patient may make his selection of **the annexed formulæ.**

Caustic Injection.

Nitrate of Silver, 4 grains; Water, 1 ounce. *Mix.*

Sulphate of Zinc and Tannin Injection.

Sulphate of Zinc, 8 grains; Tannin, 1 scruple; Water, **5** ounces. *Mix.*

Chloride of Zinc Injection.

Chloride of Zinc, 6 grains; **Soft Water, 2 ounces.** *Mix.*—**This is very ser-viceable** in obstinate cases.

Tonic Drops.

Take of Tincture of Sesquichloride of Iron, ½ ounce; Disulphate of Iron, 30 grains; Tincture of Cantharides, 1 drachm; Distilled Water, 3 ounces; Simple Syrup, ½ **ounce.** *Mix.*—Take **a** teaspoonful twice daily in a little water.

Turpentine Pills.

Pills made of Canada Turpentine, rolled up with liquorice powder. Two, three, or four, may be taken twice daily.

Tonic Pills.

This is a very nice pill. Take of Sulphate of Iron, Composition Kino Pow-der, **Venice Turpentine,** Extract of Gentian, **each** ½ drachm. *Mix.* and di-**vide into 24 pills. Take 1,** two, three or four times, daily.

Aperient Pills.

During the persistence of Tonic and stimulating medicines, the bowels may be kept open by any mild laxative. The following pill or pills will do. Take **of** Compound Rhubarb Pills, 5 grains each.—1 or 2 for a dose.

CHANGING THE REMEDIES.

Upon the principles of *"trying something else"* is often advantageous ; for it is useless repeating what has been found unsuccessful ; and it is folly to throw up our endeavors, particularly when it is shown the disease rarely cures itself.

If the Gleet proceed from disordered or acrid urine, the attention must be directed to that secretion. The drinks, and diet, as in the earlier stages of Gonorrhœa, must be adhered to. The warm bath and rest must come in also for a share of the treatment. Where there is reason to believe that general debility prevails, that the bodily health is enfeebled, that the patient has become Hypochondriacal, it is most admirable to try change of air and scene.

STRICTURE OF THE URETHRA.

Of all diseases of the genito-urinary system, stricture must be allowed to be the most terrible. It is not the most difficult to cure ; but it involves, when neglected, more serious disturbances —disturbances which frequently terminate only with loss of life. Stricture is a disease unfortunately of extensive prevalence ; and in nine cases out of ten is, the sequence of local irritation, consequent generally upon Gonorrhœa or Gleet. The first indications are the lengthened time required in urinating, the act is not performed so cleanly as it used to be; the stream differs in its flow, seldom comes out full and free, but generally split into three or four fountain-like spirts.

At other times, it twists into a spiral form, and then suddenly splits into two or more streams, whilst at the same moment the urine drops over the person or clothes, unless great care be observed.

In advanced cases, the urethra becomes so narrow, and the bladder so loses its power to expel the urine forward, that it then falls upon the shoes or trousers, or between them.

In the next attack which is very difficult to avert, the patient finds that he cannot, complete the act of making water without several interruptions, and each attended with a painful desire resembling that induced by too long retention of that fluid.

Fig. 42.

With respect to the change consequent upon permanent stricture, dissection enables us in some degree to arrive at the truth. Excrescences and tubercles have been found growing from the wall of the urethra; but in the majority of instances, the only perceptible change is a thickening of the canal here and there of indefinite length ; but whether it be occasioned by the exudation of coagulable lymph, or whether it be the adhesion of ulcerated surfaces, which I contend are more or less present in Gleet, is not so easy to determine : at all events it is undoubtedly the result of inflammation of the urethra.

Spasmodic Stricture is generally seated at the neck of the

bladder, and may occur to persons in good health from exposure
to wet or cold; from some digestive derangement; from long
retention of urine, particularly while walking, owing to the
absence of public urinals; or to violent horse-exercise; but more
frequently does it happen to those young men who, when suffering
from Gleet or Gonorrhœa, imperfectly or perfectly cured, commit
excesses in diet or drink. Stricture may also be caused by injuries,
by falling, blows, wounds, and also by masturbation.

The following diagrams are further explanatory of stricture in its
amplified forms.

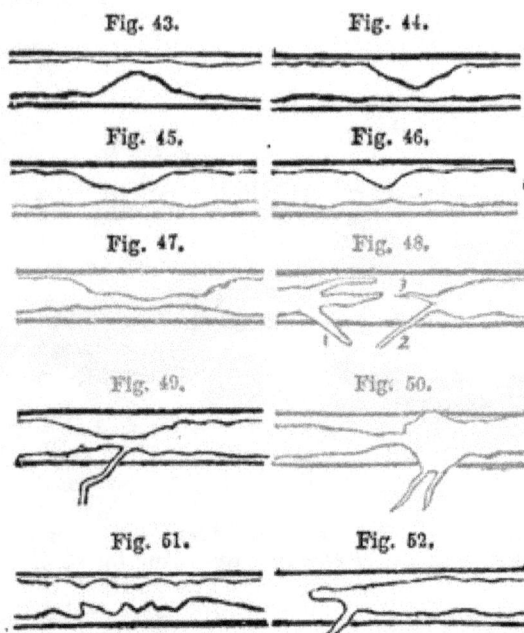

Fig. 43.   Fig. 44.

Fig. 45.   Fig. 46.

Fig. 47.   Fig. 48.

Fig. 49.   Fig. 50.

Fig. 51.   Fig. 52.

The dark marginal lines denote the calibre of the urethra, and
the thin inner lines the actual diameter of the obstructed passage.
Fig. 43 shows the stricture to be on the upper part of the urethra.
Fig. 44, the lower part.   Fig. 45, exhibits a stricture of some
length, and a somewhat contracted state of the whole canal. Fig.
46 denotes a very common form of stricture, which resembles a
bag tied in the middle; it is the least difficult to cure of any,
because it signifies that the seat of irritation is limited; but these
cases are generally precursory to severer forms, if not promptly
attended to. Fig. 47 represents a stricture of considerable length,
and of course very difficult of removal.

The clumsy introduction of a bougie, or, in other instances,
the unjustifiable introduction of one, is likely to, and very frequently does, lacerate the delicate and irritable membrane, and
make a false passage. Fig. 48 exhibits an instance in 1 and 2;

the upper numerical shows a false passage made by a bougie, and an obliteration of the ordinary passage of the urethra, the result of inflammation, constituting an impassable stricture; the lower figure exhibits a false opening made, in the first instance, by a fruitless effort at passing an instrument, when inflammation completed the process. No urine escaped from it, of course; because communication was cut off from the bladder by the impassable stricture, the outlet for the discharge of that fluid being through a sinuous opening marked 2; 3 denoting the closed end of the urethra. Fig. 49 exhibits a stricture, where the posture part was enlarged by the constant pressure of the urine to escape through the narrowed part of the urethra; ulceration ensued, and a fistulous opening was the consequence; the stricture was seated high up, and the fistulous canal was several inches long, terminating in the upper and posterior part of the thigh; the urine used to dribble through it as well as through the urethra. In Fig. 50 is presented an illustration of extensive ulceration producing two fistulous openings: the state of the urethra was only discovered after death. Fig. 51 portrays irregular and extensive ulceration. Fig. 52 shows an impervious urethra, and a fistulous opening, through which the urine flowed.

TREATMENT.

Stricture, if early attended to, is a disease easily remediable; if neglected, its horrors accumulate, and sufferings the most acute close the scene. Such, however, is the process of science, that it is almost possible to cure the most inveterate case—at all events, to relieve it; but that is no reason why the initiatory notices should be disregarded. Stricture is of two kinds, spasmodic and permanent: the treatment of the first is chiefly medical, the treatment of the latter chiefly mechanical. The principal agents I rely upon, in the cure of the former, are the warm bath, rest, sedatives, and certain dietetic restrictions: for the removal of the latter I place unbounded confidence in the practice of *dilatation*.

One of the most powerful adjuncts in the treatment of all affections of the urethra, bladder, prostate gland, kidneys and other structures, pertaining to the urinary and generative system, is the warm bath.

The only mode of ascertaining the precise condition of the urethra is by an examination of it, which should not be delayed a moment after suspicion is entertained of the impending evil.

The cure of dilatation is as follows:—The seat of the stricture being ascertained, a bougie, somewhat larger than the calibre of the urinary current, warmed and dipped in an oleaginous mixture, combined with some sedative or stimulant, according to circumstances, is to be passed to the stricture, and the gentlest pressure employed for the space of five, ten, or twelve minutes, according to the irritation it produces, removing it as soon as any uneasiness is felt.

The bougie, is to be pressed softly, but steadily against the obstruction, now and then withholding for a minute the bearing, so as to allow a respite to the stretched membrane; the renewing, by what is better done than expressed, an "insinuating" pressure for the space of time advised above. The patient should not be dispirited even if the bougie do not perforate the stricture at the first trial; it would doubtless do so, if longer time were employed but that is rarely advisable, except in cases where the urine can scarcely escape, or much expedition be requisite. Should the operation even be unsuccessful in the first attempt, the patient will find his ability to micturate much greater than before the introduction. A great advantage of the cure by dilatation, independently of its safety and efficacy, is the insignificant pain it occasions; the sensation produced being only like a pressing desire to make water, which immediately subsides on withdrawing the bougie.

An entrance having been gained, a bougie of a larger size is selected on the next occasion, and the same process repeated. It is seldom advisable to repeat the operation oftener than once in two days, except in cases of great urgency, and when the urethra is irritable, only every three or four days.

Fig. 53.

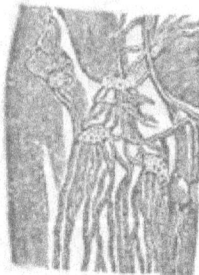

THE INGENUAL GLANDS and the absorbents showing their communication and Nature.

By continuing in this manner, the stricture gradually yields, and a bougie, as large as the orifice will permit to enter, will at last proceed through the whole passage without meeting with any obstacle. The operation should not be wholly laid aside, but continued until the disposition for contraction is entirely removed: and the patient should occasionally examine his urethra, every month or two, lest he encounter a relapse.

SYPHILIS OR POX.

Syphilis is another and more violent form of the venereal disease then Gouorrhœa. It is characterized by the appearance of a pimple surrounded by a slight inflammation, and the formation of an ulcer or chancre. The ulcer generally appears in from five to fourteen days after exposure.

Chancres are of different varieties, and may be very destructive to the organ, and there is generally a bubo or swelling in the groin, which appears in a few days after the ulcer; this swelling may continue until matter forms, when it may break, or require to be opened.

When syphilis affects the constitution, it is known as secondary, and tertiary; it then shows itself in the forms of eruptions, sore throat, and ulcers in different parts of the body.

The eruption generally appears on the forehead, back, legs and arms, copper colored, attended with slight itching; the pustule is sometimes filled with a pale fluid. When the mouth and throat are affected, the parts become swollen and sore, or red and covered with a white membrane, or there may be a pale yellow ulcer of the throat or tonsils, or a dark, livid, and sloughing ulcer, which may extend to the various parts about the throat, and nose, destroying the bones of the face.

TREATMENT.

As soon as the ulcer appears on the penis, it should be immediately touched with caustic. The caustics which may be used are Nitrate of Silver, Nitric Acid, Caustic Potassa, Chloride of Zinc. The Nitrate of Silver is the most used, and the pimple should be thoroughly burned. After the sore has been cauterized, a piece of lint dipped in a solution of opium, in the proportion of one drachm of opium, to four ounces of water, should be laid upon it, and the penis enveloped in a piece of muslin and covered with oiled silk.

Fig. 54.

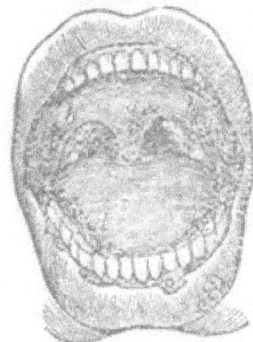

ULCERATION of the throat or palate by the venereal virus.

The following solution may be used, instead of the Opium :

Salphate of Copper, 1 grain; Water 1 ounce. This should be applied frequently, and the parts washed twice a day with castile soap and water.

The following may be taken internally :

Protiodide of Mercury, 12 grains ; Conserve of Roses, 1 scruple. Divide into twelve or twenty-four pills, and take one twice a day.

The following may be used with advantage in some cases :

Blue Pill, ½ drachm; Extract of Henbane, 1 scruple. Make into ten pills. Dose, one pill at night.

Or this

Corrosive Sublimate, 4 grains; Extract of Opium, 5 grains. Mix—and make into twenty pills. Dose, one pill night and morning.

These preparations of Mercury should not be used more than five days in succession, as there is danger of producing salivation. If salivation is produced, use the following :

Chlorinated Soda, 1 ounce: Water, 2 ounces. Mix.—The mouth should be rinsed out with this several times a day, being careful not to swallow any of it.

Ricord reccommends Iron to be given in the proportion of one part of the Potassio-Tartrate of Iron, to six parts of water. Two teaspoonfuls given three times a day. The same preparation should be applied to the sore. The bubo or swelling in the groin, should be treated with compression. If, however, matter forms, the sore should be opened and poulticed. In case of an eruption on the skin, or when the disease shows itself in the throat or other part of the body, the Iodide of Potassium may be given as follows :

Compound Infusion of Sarsaparilla, 1 pint; Iodide of Potassium, 1½ ounce; Mix—Dose, a teaspoonful after every meal.

The Preparation called Donovan's Solution, may be given internally, in doses of from three to five drops.

The diet should be strictly regular, the patient not being allowed to eat any stimulating food, or drink liquors.

CHAPTER XV.

SELF-ABUSE—NOCTURNAL EMISSIONS—IMPOTENCE—STERILITY.

Few are aware of the extent to which self-pollution is practiced by the young of both sexes in civilized society, and none but those whose position or professional confidence brings them into advisory and intimate relations with the victims of unnatural indulgences or venereal excesses can have an adequate conception of the evils resulting therefrom. None but the medical man can trace the deplorable consequences to feeble, malformed, puny, and imperfectly organized offspring, and no one but the physiologist can clearly see all the external marks of exhausted vitality and premature decay stamped indelibly on thousands of our young men and maidens otherwise in the bloom of youth, health and beauty.

We might fill a volume with instances of the effects of this baneful habit, and a mere enumeration of the diseases directly or indirectly induced by these practices would occupy a far larger space than can be allowed. We shall, therefore, simply show the direct effects of the habit, and give plain and specific directions for the cure.

The abuse of amativeness rapidly exhausts the nervous power, the generative function, and takes strength from the organic and animal powers. If it fail all fail. The stomach cannot digest for want of the nervous energy spent in oft repeated and fruitless orgasms. Nutrition cannot be carried on in the capillary system. The waste matter, which should be carried off by the secreting and excreting organs, is retained to poison the fountains of life. The skin becomes dry and withered, the eye dull, the mind weak and disordered, all noble passions lose their force, the whole system is in discord and disorder, and ready to become a prey to disease. Then comes epilepsy, spinal disease, dropsy, or some form of consumption.

The genital organs are, as it were, woven into the same grand web of organic life with the stomach, heart, lungs, etc., by being largely supplied with the same class of nerves on which the organs of nutrition depend for their functional power; but the genital organs are also supplied with nerves of animal life, or those which are connected with the brain and spinal marrow. Hence the influences of the brain may act directly on the genital organs; and of these latter, on the brain. Lascivious thoughts and imaginations will excite and stimulate the genital organs, cause an increased quantity of blood to flow into them, and augment their secretions and peculiar sensibilities; and, on the other hand, the excited state of the genital organs, either from the stimulations of semen or from diseased action in the system, will throw its influence upon the brain, and force lascivious thoughts and imaginations upon the mind.

It is supposed by many that the mischief of this practice is from loss of semen. The loss of this secretion is certainly exhausting, but is far from being the greatest evil. Boys secrete no semen before puberty, and girls never secrete any. The real source of mischief is the nervous orgasm—that vivid, ecstatic, and, in its natural exercise, most delightful of sensuous enjoyments. The orgasm is almost a spasm, when prematurely excited, and though then imperfect it gives a shock to the whole system, and when often repeated the nervous power is completely exhausted. All the vitality of the body goes to supply the immature and exhausted amative organism; the brain and body.

The following are given by reputable medical writers as some of the effects of this baneful habit.

Loss of memory and mental power; entire concentration of imagination on one feeling or act; a besotted, embarrassed, melancholy, and stupid look; loss of presence of mind; incapability of bearing the gaze of any one; tremors and apprehensions of future misery; morbid appetite; indigestion, and the whole train of dyspeptic symptoms; constipation; foetid breath, etc.; pale, sallow, cadaverous, or greasy-looking skin; eruptions over the face; hollowness, and lack of lustre in the eyes, with a dark circle around them; feebleness of the whole body; indisposition to make any exertion; weakness, weariness, and dull pain in the small of the back; creeping sensation in the spine; finally there comes insanity or idiocy, or atrophy and death by consumption.

Self-pollution is the most certain, though not always the most immediate and direct avenue to destruction. It constitutes a lingering species of mortality, and if it were possible to study and invent refinement in cruelty, surely that would most clearly deserve the designation, which a man points deliberately against himself—against not merely his temporal but external welfare; not by sudden wrench to tear himself away from the amenities of wife, children, and home, but with his own hand imperceptibly to infuse a deadly poison, slowly to rankle in the cup of life and embitter each passing day; to shroud in gloom the darkening future, and invite the king of terrors prematurely to do his office.

A youth endowed by Nature with talent and genius becomes dull or totally stupid; the mind loses all relish for virtuous or exalted ideas; the consciousness of the purity and essential holiness of the Creator, operates as a bar against any approach to him, or the appropriation of any of those consolations under suffering which religion is destined to afford.

All his fire and spirit are deadened by this detestible vice; he is like a faded rose, a tree blasted in its bloom, a wandering skeleton; nothing remains but debility, languor, livid paleness, a withered body, and a degraded soul. The whole life of such a man is a continued succession of secret reproach, painful sensations, arising from the consciousness of having been the fabricator of his own distress, irresolution, disgust of life, and not unfrequently self-murder. Nay, what in effect is this but the consummation of slow self-destruction? Could we but lift the veil of the grave, how should we startle at the long train of the victims of sensualism?

The first step to be taken for the cure of these sad effects is at once and forever abandon the filthy habit. There must be no indecision here, no temporizing—it must be broken off at once, · and then by attention to a strict hygienic regimen a cure will be effected.

The only power on earth by which the deceased and disordered body can possibly regain health is by Nature's own renovating process, which sometimes seems to work slow, and for a long time to make no progress. If the system is very much reduced and the patient afflicted with involuntary nocturnal emissions, and distressed with pains, and impaired senses, and enfeebled mind, and cheerless melancholy, tending to despair and madness, he must remember the general and special sympathies and reciprocities which exist between the genital organs and the alimentary canal and the brain; and remember, too, that in this morbid and exceedingly excitable and irritable condition of the system, things which may seem too trifling to deserve notice may, nevertheless, be sufficient to keep up the disorders of the body, and therefore it is hardly possible to be too cautious, while in this condition, in regard to everything which concerns regimen and conduct. Every irritation, every undue excitement of the brain, stomach, and intestines, is calculated to continue the involuntary emissions; while the latter, in turn, keep up and increase the morbid irritability of those organs. Improper quantities of the best aliment in nature will produce the same effect; and so also will the presence of food in the stomach, deodenum, etc., at improper times. An over-fulness, or late supper, will almost invariably cause this evil in those who are liable to such an affliction; and while those emissions continue, it is impossible for the system to recover strength and health. Costiveness of the bowels is also sure to keep up the nightly discharges; and if recourse be had to medicine, for the purpose of keeping the bowels open, it is sure to perpetuate the mischief, by irritating and debilitating still more the tissues of the alimentary canal, and, through them, the whole system.

The food, therefore, must be of such a character as will pass through the stomach and intestines with the least irritation and oppression, while it at the same time affords sufficient nourishment, and causes a free and healthy action of the bowels. Farinaceous food, properly prepared, is incomparably the best aliment, and good bread, made of coarsely ground, unbolted wheat, rye, or Indian corn, is also admitted to be one of the very best articles of diet that can be used.

When the nightly emissions are frequent, and the system very much irritated, the patient should confine himself to a few articles of diet, and eat but little, carefully avoiding full and late suppers. No animal food should be used at all, and no other drink but pure water should be ever drank.

Many young men, by observing these rules, have been entirely relieved from emissions, but on drinking a single glass of wine, brandy-and-water, or malt liquors, or a cup of coffee, or eating a full meal, it would cause the emissions to come on again the succeeding night. The patient cannot be too careful to observe a strict, undeviating regimen, and to scrupulously avoid spirits, wine, malt liquors, and every kind of alcoholic drink, even in the smallest quantity; and opium, tobacco, coffee, tea, and all other narcotics; and pepper, ginger, mustard, horse-radish, peppermint, and, in short, every kind of stimulating and heating substance.

If the patient requires something more warming and stimulating than farinaceous food and water, to increase the tone and action of the organs, and enable them to perform their functions satisfactorily, he should not use stimulants, which, while they increase the action, necessarily deteriorate the functional results, and impair the vital properties of the tissues on which they act, especially when there are natural, healthy and invigorating means of increasing the tone and action of his organs, and general vigor of his system, by active exercise. Let him exhilarate himself by free and copious draughts of the pure air of heaven. Let him go to the gymnasium and with moderate beginning, and moderate increase of effort, let him swing upon and climb the poles, the ropes and ladders, and vault upon the wooden horse and practice all the other feats of that admirable institution; or let him walk and run and jump, or labor on the farm; and avoid sedentary habits, and all anxieties and excitements of the mind; and most strictly shun all dalliance with females, and all lewd books, and obscene conversation and lascivious images and thoughts. Let him sleep on a hard bed, and rise early in the morning and take a shower bath of cold water, or plunge into cold water, or sponge his body all over with it; and, in either case rub himself off briskly and freely with a good stiff flesh-brush; and then exercise vigorously in the open air, or in the gymnasium, for an hour before breakfast. Let him exercise as much as he can through the day; let him take an early, light supper, and take a good deal of active exercise before going to bed; and, if his nocturnal emissions still continue, let him just before getting into bed, repeat his shower or sponge or sitz bath, and follow it freely with the coarse towel.

Let him perseveringly observe this regimen, without the slightest deviation in a single instance, and let him increase his exercise with his increasing strength—avoiding constantly an excess of aliment; and after awhile his nocturnal emissions and other disorders will disappear and his strength and general vigor will increase, and he will become cheerful and sprightly, and feel as if new life and new hopes were dawning on him; and when he is fully established in these improvements, he may gradually relax the rigor of his diet, and take a greater variety of simple vegetables and fruits; but still he had better never go beyond the vegetable kingdom and pure water for his aliment.

By these means—if by any, short of miraculous power—and by these alone, can the unhappy sufferer hope to be restored to comfortable and permanent health and enjoyment. The progress will be slow, but incomparably the safest and surest; and health restored in this way will put his body in a condition which will, in the greatest degree, secure it from future prostration and suffering, and from transmitting the evils of his former errors to an innocent and helpless progeny.

SEMINAL EMISSIONS.

There are few diseases whose victims are in a more pitiable condition than those who suffer from seminal losses. Very many cases have come under our observation, and the following advice, when faithfully followed, has been attended with benefit.

The general trouble—loss of semen, and consequent exhaustion—takes place under several different circumstances. In some cases, the seminal loss is attended by a voluptuous dream. Such dreams occur to passionate persons of both sexes. Where this action occurs but seldom, and in consequence of the accumulation of vital power in this part of the organism, it cannot be a source of any great mischief, though a poor substitute for the natural gratification of amative desire, but in men, in certain states of the system, there comes on an excessive excitability or irritability of the organs, which makes these dreams occur with exhausting frequency. The semen is continually voided, with a ruinous expenditure of nervous power. The seminal vesicles are irritated by the presence of the smallest quantity of the fluid; the nervous action is excited, and the exhaustion follows. It is difficult for any well man to conceive of the weak, hopeless, miserable, despairing condition of the victim to this disease. He feels coming upon him all the consequences of masturbation, without having the power to prevent them. The habit is not within his volition. The nervous organism is performing for itself what the voluntary muscles perform for the victim of solitary vice. Hundreds of young men are driven to suicide by this disease—hundreds more drown the sense of suffering by the excesses of dissipation. All hope of genial life is destroyed. There is no love, no marriage, no children, no ambition—for all power of mind and body is wasted. In some cases, the action seems confined to the spinal centre—the cerebellum no longer acts. The semen is voided unconsciously. Sometimes, in extreme cases, it oozes away without erection, or the slightest sensation of pleasure, even passing off with the urine.

Masturbation is the cause of this terrible disease, in nine cases in ten. When the victim of this diseased habit would stop, he finds that a fiend has taken the place of his volition; a fiend he has raised but cannot quell. Continence is sometimes supposed to be a cause, such cases however, are extremely doubtful. All diseasing and debilitating influences may co-operate in causing this condition. Exhaustion, even by natural means, especially in promiscuous or unloving unions, may bring on the irritability or weakness. Married men have it occasionally, as well as single. There is no more potent cause than tobacco; and the whole class of nervous stimulants favor this action. It is only a particular direction of what we call nervousness.

The weakness may also result from worms in the rectum. It may be known by an itching near the base of the penis. These may readily be removed by injections of warm water. As much water should be thrown up as the rectum will hold, and this must be allowed to descend suddenly, when it will wash out whatever worms that may be within reach of the water.

In regard to the cure, there is but two or three directions to be given, beside those already given for the cure of masturbation. Let the patient, in all respects, as far as possible, place himself in the conditions of health. Let him regulate his food by his digestion, carefully evacuate his bowels every night, sleep cool, and before going to bed take a sitz-bath, beginning at a temperature of ninety degrees. Day after day cool gradually, at the rate of one degree a day. In this way you will moderate the action of the parts, and allay the irritability. Cold water may be applied night and morning to the cerebellum. In the morning take a full bath of cold water, and a thorough rubbing. As the cure progresses, the patient will have his sitz-bath colder, and may apply other means of invigoration, as dashing cold water upon the genitals, the rising douche, etc., use also the following tonic:

Sulphate of Quinine, 15 grains ; Diluted Sulphuric Acid. 15 drops ; Compound Tincture of Cardamons. 3 drachms, Tincture of Hops, 3 drachms; Compound Infusion of Roses. 6 ounces. Mix.—Dose. one or two tablespoonfuls in a wine glass of water, two or three times a day.

This also has produced excellent results.

Rose Water, 6 ounces: Syrup of Orange peel, 1 ounce; Muriated Tincture of Iron, 1 ounce. Mix.—Dose, one teaspoonful in a wine glass of water, after each meal.

Several appliances are sold for the purpose of stopping these emissions; they are generally a ring, modified more or less, that is placed on the penis when in a quiet state, so that its erection and enlargement cannot take place without awaking the patient from the pressure of the ring. These contrivances are to be avoided. They cannot do good, and may cause much injury to the urethra and seminal ducts.

By persistently following this treatment, a cure is certain. In most cases no medicines of any kind are required and the cure is in the patient's own hands. Strict attention to the laws of health, morally and physically, is all that is necessary to effect a complete and permanent cure. Sufferers from this infirmity are generally too anxious about symptoms, they are continually watching and fretting about the urine, urinary pains, etc., and excited and nervous imagination magnifying ordinary trifles into serious and alarming indications. The best plan is to pay no attention to these matters whatever. If any symptom is very alarming, application to the family physician or any respectable practitioner would set matters right. Marriage has been recommended as a cure for seminal weakness, but it more frequently aggravates and increases the disease. Before the marriage relation is entered into the health should be fully restored.

IMPOTENCE AND STERILITY.

Impotence is an absolute cause of sterility, because it prevents the conditions necessary to fecundation from taking place ; but although the act of coitus may be accomplished, it does not follow "that the person should always be able to perpetuate his species. Stricture of the urethra may prevent the discharge of seminal fluid; or the fluid may be directed towards the bladder or the parietes of the urethra, by deviation of the orifices of the ejaculatory ducts. The secretion may be altered in its nature, it may only contain imperfect spermatozoa, etc. A man may, therefore, be unfruitful without being impotent.

Masturbation leads directly to impotence in men and women, and often to sterility in the former. Barrenness in women is not as in men, the result of impotence. The organs, external and internal, may loose their sensibility to pleasure and still the ovaries may form their germs and the uterus may nourish them. Barrenness in women may proceed from falling or other displacement of the womb ; from the closing of its mouth ; from leucorrhœa or whites, or other diseased discharge, which may arrest and destroy the zoospermes; or it may be caused by inflammation, or excessive irritability of the uterus, by which the embryos are thrown off in a series of early abortions, and the same result may be produced by the frequent excitement of amativeness.

The cure of sterility in men in those rare cases in which it exists without impotence, must come with health. Use the same treatment as for masturbation.

The cure of impotence must be a course of gradual invigoration. Put the patient into the best of possible healthy conditions, and the cure will come.

In addition to these means, the following may be taken :

Hoxham's Tincture of Cinchona, 4 ounces; Diluted Phosphoric Acid, ½ ounce; Tincture of Nux Vomica, 2 drachms. *Miz.*—Dose, 1 teaspoonful every 3 hours.

The impotence of women requires corresponding treatment, with bathing, the sitz-bath, the wet bandage and the vagina syringe. Take also the following pills:

Citrate of Iron, 1 drachm; Sulphate of Quinine, 1 scruple; Extract of Nux Vomica, 8 grains. *Miz.*—Make into 32 pills. Dose 1 pill three times a day.

But when barrenness comes from excessive action, it must be treated like nymphomania.

Nymphomania in women, and Satyriasis in men, are the names given to inflamed and excited conditions of the generative function. The seats of this disease are in the cerebellum, extending to the whole brain and involving every feeling; the lower part of the spinal cord, exciting continual erections and automatic and spasmodic action; and the generative organs.

Its causes are masturbation; exciting diet; an indolent, sensual and voluptuous life; and continence, or forced abstinence from the enjoyments of love.

The symptoms of this disease are an excessive and perpetual desire for sexual intercourse, a mind filled with lascivious ideas, and excited to frenzy by every voluptuous image. There is no longer any discrimination of beauty, fitness or attraction to the diseased man every female, and even a female animal, is an object of desire. Under its influence men have committed rapes on little children and aged women, and committed other vile abominations.

When women or girls are effected with nymphomania, there are similar and even more striking manifestations.

When the disease is brought on by masturbation, the habit must of course be at once broken off and some active occupation be engaged in to engage and absorb the whole energies of body and mind.

A spare and entirely unstimulating diet, the sitz-bath, the cold douche, or ice-water to the cerebellum, are plainly indicated. The vagina syringe helps to overcome the inflammation of the womb, and the wet bandage, often renewed, should be worn around the loins by women, and should cover the genital organs in men. The treatment is, in fact, very similar to that for masturbation, or inflammation of any other part of the system.

CHAPTER XVI.

DISEASES PECULIAR TO WOMEN.

DELAYED AND OBSTRUCTED MENSTRUATION.

When the menses do not appear at the time when they may naturally be expected, we call it delayed or obstructed menstruation. It is, however, of great importance to know whether a girl is sufficiently developed to make it necessary for the menses to appear, although she may have reached the proper age. As long as the girl has not increased physically, if she has not become wider across the hips, if her breasts have not become enlarged, and if she experience none of the changes incident to this period, an effort to force nature is positively injurious. In this case a general treatment will be called for. She should be required to exercise freely in the open air, retire early to bed, and arise at an early hour in the morning. She should not be allowed to be closely confined at school, if attending. Her diet should be generous, but free from all rich food, which will disorder the stomach. If, however, she is fully developed, and she suffers from time to time from congestions of the head, breast, or abdomen, it will be necessary to interfere. The following are the symptoms which will generally be found in these cases : Headache, weight, fullness, and throbbing in the centre of the cranium, and in the back part of the head; pains in the back and loins; cold feet and hands, becoming sometimes very hot ; skin harsh and dry ; slow pulse, and not unfrequently attended with epilepsy.

TREATMENT.

It is well for the patient, a few days before the period, to take a warm hip or foot bath twice a day, and at night when retiring to apply cloths wet in warm water to the lower part of the abdomen.

The bowels should be kept open, by some mild cathartic as castor oil, or a pill of Aloes. If there is pain and fullness of the head during the discharge, or before it, use the following :

Tincture of Aconite Leaves, 2 drachms; Tincture of Belladonna, 1 drachm; Tincture of Cantharides, 1 drachm ; Morphia, 3 grains ; Simple Syrup, 4 ounces. Dose—one teaspoonful three times a day. If the pain is severe it may be taken every two hours.

Between the periods, if the system is weak, the following may be taken :

Procip. Carbonate of Iron, 5 drachms; Extract Conium, 2 drachms; Balsam Peru, 1 drachm; Alcohol, 4 ounces; Oil Wintergreen, 20 drops; Simple Syrup, 8 ounces. Dose—two teaspoonfuls three times a day. Shake the mixture before using.

CHLOROSIS OR GREEN SICKNESS.

This disease generally occurs in young unmarried females, who are weak and delicate. It manifests itself about the age of puberty, and is accompanied by feeble appetite, and digestion. There is no menstrual discharge, or else it is very slight.

It is caused by unnutricious food, residence in damp and ill-ventilated apartments. It may be hereditary, all the females of the family being liable to the same disease. Those who drink largely of tea, coffee, diluted acids, bad wines, and indulge in tight lacing, are predisposed to this disease. Among the exciting causes may be mentioned disturbing emotions, unrequited love, home sickness, depression of spirits, &c.

If we take into consideration the fact that the cause of the disease is impoverishment of the blood, the treatment will not be difficult. Exercise freely in the open air; protect the body from chilliness by warm clothing, and plenty of it. The patient should sleep on a mattrass, in a well ventilated room. The diet should be nourishing, without being stimulating. It is important that the habits should be regular, and the mind kept cheerful by society and innocent amusements. Before the medical treatment is commenced, the exciting causes of the disease must be removed. A complete change must be made in the existence of the patient. If she is confined closely at school, she must be removed; if she is inclined to confine herself to the house, send her to the country. Picture to her the danger she is in, by the continuance of such a life; give her plenty of out-door exercise. The mental and moral causes are the most difficult to remove, but a change of scenery and new friends will do much towards it. For those who are shut up in factories, or who work all day in a stooping position, a change of employment must be made. A bath of tepid water in the morning followed by a brisk rubbing will be beneficial. Also the frequent use of the sitting bath, and the sponge bath in the evening. Active exercise should precede and follow all baths. During menstruation all applications of water should be omitted.

The following receipes are recommended by Dr. Pancoast, of Philadelphia. They are to be taken on alternate days; that is, take No. 1 on one day, No. 2 the next day, and so on:

No. 1.—Precip. Carbonate of Iron, 5 drachms; Extract of Conium, 2 drachms; Balsam Peru, 1 drachm; Oil Cinnamon, 20 drops; Simple Syrup, 8 ounces; Pulverized Gum Arabic, 2 drachms. *Mix.*—Dose, two teaspoonfuls three times a day, every other day after meals. Shake before using.

No. 2.—Tincture of Nux Vomica, 1 drachm; Syrup Iodide of Iron, 1 ounce; Simple Syrup, 4 ounces. *Mix.*—Dose one teaspoonful three times a day, every other day, in water after meals. Another treatment is as follows:

Clear the bowels with the following mixture:

Sulphate of Magnesia, 1 ounce; Nitrate of Potash, 10 grains; Extract of Liquorice, 1 scruple; Compound Infusion of Senna, 5½ ounces; Tincture of Jalap, 3 drachms; Spirit of Sal Volatile, 1 drachm. *Mix.*—Dose two or three tablespoonfuls at a time, at intervals of two hours, until an effect is produced.

This is to be followed by Sulphate of Iron, 5 grains; Extract of Gentian, 10 grains. Make into three pills, and take a pill twice a day, with the Compound Aloes or Rhubarb pill every night.

PROFUSE MENSTRUATION—MENORRHAGIA.

By Menorrhagia we understand an immoderate flow of the menses. There is no fixed amount of blood which is lost at the menstrual period, but it varies in different women. It will average, however, from four to eight ounces. The quantity discharged may be estimated by the number of napkins used. Each napkin will contain about half an ounce, or one tablespoonful, so that eight napkins would contain four ounces; twenty, ten ounces, etc. In some females the discharge may be excessive, without impairment of the general health.

Some females are predisposed to uterine hemorrhages, from a relaxed, or flabby state of the texture of the uterus. Frequent child-bearing, abortion, high living, too prolonged and frequent suckling, may **induce flooding**. Among the exciting causes we may mention, over-exertion, dancing, falls, lifting heavy weights, cold, and mental excitements.

TREATMENT.

The patient must lie down on a hard bed, and abstain from all stimulating food and drinks. The room should be cool, and she should be lightly covered with bed clothes. Soak the feet in warm water, and if the flowing is excessive apply **cloths**, wrung out in vinegar and water, to the lower bowels. The hips must be elevated higher than the head. Only in extreme **cases** should plugging be resorted to. This may be done by pieces **of linen**, about four inches square, **thrust into** the vagina, until **it is full, and a** bandage applied between **the legs.** Cold hip baths, **and vaginal** injections of cold **water will be beneficial** when the hemorrhage is slight.

Use also the following:

Diluted Sulphuric Acid, 2 drachms; Syrup of Orange-Peel 2 ounces; Cinnamon Water, 1 ounce. *Mix.*—Dose, a teaspoonful in a wine-glass of water, two or three times a day.

If there is much pain administer the following every two or three hours:

Morphia, ¼ grain; Cayenne, 4 grains; Rosin, 4 grains, *Mix.*—Give in Blackberry Syrup.

PAINFUL MENSTRUATION—MENSTRUAL COLIC— DYSMENORRHŒA.

The word *dysmenorrhœa* means a difficult monthly flow, and is always preceded by severe pains in the back and lower part of the abdomen. **It is caused by** taking **cold** during the period; fright, violent **mental emotions;** obstinate constipation; sedentary occupations; **smallness of the mouth and** neck **of the** womb. Females subject to this trouble are generally relieved by marriage. The symptoms are severe bearing down pains in the region of the uterus like labor pains; restlessness, coldness, flashes of heat, with headache; aching in the small of the back, lower part of the abdomen, and thighs; the discharge is scanty, and contains shreds of fibre and clotted blood.

TREATMENT.

The patient should **immediately go to** bed, and cover up warmly. Stimulating food **and** drinks **should be** avoided. Use a warm foot bath and sitting bath, with hot poultices **of hops, or cloths, wet** in hot water applied to the abdomen.

In the interval of **the menses**, take active exercise, with a tepid hip bath, three nights in the week, injecting some of the water high up into the vagina. **Keep the bowels open with a pill** of Aloes **and Myrrh, and take a small** teaspoonful of the volatile Tincture of Guaicum, three times a day in water. On the approach of the period, take the following, at night:

Calomel, 3 grains; Opium, 1 grain. In the morning, a dose of Castor Oil, and on the appearance of the menses, tho Dover's Powder, and mixture, as before. Repeat this treatment in each interval, until permanently relieved.

The following is recommended by Prof. **Meigs**, to be taken a few days before the period :

Acetous Tincture of Colchicum, 3 drachms; Magnesia, 1 drachm; Sulphate of Magnesia, 3 drachms Distilled Mint, or Cinnamon Water, 4 ounces. *Mix.* —Dose, a small wineglassful every two or three hours, until it operates. **This** should be preceded, the night before, by a small dose of blue pill.

SUPPRESSION OF THE MENSES, (*Amenorrhœa.*)

By suppression is meant a disappearance of the menses, after they have become established, and may be either acute or chronic. It is caused by cold, caught during the flow, by exposure to night air, or by wetting the feet, fear, shocks, violent mental emotions, anxiety, fevers, and other acute diseases. Chronic suppression may be either a consequence of the acute, or caused by delicate health; also from diseases of the ovaries, or womb. It may also be occasioned by an imperforate hymen, in which case it must be cut open by a physician.

When the suppression is caused by some disease in the system, that disease must be cured before the menses will return. For sudden suppression, use the warm sitting bath or foot bath. Apply cloths wet in warm water to the lower part of the abdomen, and drink freely of warm water. If the suppression is chronic, and the patient is delicate, in the interval between the menses, use the shower, or the full bath of cold or tepid water, rubbing the body briskly with a coarse towel, especially around the abdomen, loins, and genital organs.

As soon as the discharge has ceased, a warm hip bath will generally bring it on. If there is much inflammation of the uterus give the following :

Tincture Aconite leaves, 2 drachms; Sweet Spirits of Nitre, 1 ounce; Simple Syrup, 3 ounces. Dose, one teaspoonful every two or three hours.

If the discharge cannot be brought on, wait until the **next** period. A few days before the term, the bowels should be freely opened, and kept open until the period for the discharge has arrived. The pill of Aloes and Iron of the United States Dispensatory, is one of the best that can be given. Give from one to three pills daily. If there is no evident reason for the discharge not appearing, such as pregnancy, inflammation of the neck of the womb, and the woman is suffering from the suppression, use the following:

Caulophyllin, 1 drachm; Extract Aconite, 8 grains, Aloes, 10 grains; Sulphate of Iron, 10 grains. **Make into 40 pills.** Dose, two or three pills, taken night and morning.

The remedies should always be taken a few days before the period arrives for the menses. If chronic suppression is the result of any acute disease, the health must first be re-established otherwise, it would be wrong to force the menses. When this has been done, immediately before the return of the period, a warm hip bath should be taken every night for six nights, and one of the following pills taken three times a day

Fresh powdered Ergot of Rye, 50 grains; Barbadoes Aloes, 12 grains; Essential Oil of Juniper, 12 drops. Make into twelve pills, with syrup or mucilage, washing down each pill with a cupful of Pennyroyal tea.

CESSATION OF THE MENSES—CHANGE OF LIFE.

By the phrase, "change of life," or the critical period, we understand the final cessation, or stoppage of the menses. It usually takes place between the ages of forty and fifty, although in some cases it may occur as early as thirty, and in others not until sixty; however, we can expect the change about the forty-fifth year.

The symptoms will vary according to the constitution of the woman; in some the change occurs by the discharge gradually diminishing in quantity, in others by the intervals between the periods being lengthened. The woman may pass this period, without having any more unpleasant symptoms than an occasional rush of blood to the head, or a headache. Others, however, may have very severe symptoms arise, which will require the care of an intelligent physician. These disagreeable sensations should receive a careful consideration, and not be hushed up with the reply, that these complaints arise from the "change of life," and will vanish whenever that change takes place. The foundation of serious trouble may be laid, which will make the remainder of her existence a burden, and cut short a life which might have been conducted to a green old age. While this change is in progress, in probably the majority of cases, there is more or less disturbance of the health. It is sometimes quite impossible to say exactly what is the trouble with the patient, except that she is out of health. The following are some of the symptoms which may arise: Headache, dizziness, biliousness, sour stomach, indigestion, diarrhœa, costiveness, piles, itching of the private parts; cramps and colic in the bowels; palpitation of the heart; swelling of the limbs and abdomen; pains in the back and loins; paleness and general weakness.

TREATMENT.

Eat and drink moderately; sleep in airy, well ventilated rooms; avoid stimulants; exercise daily in the open air, either by walking or riding; avoid violent emotions; shun exposure to wet, stormy weather, wet feet, etc.

Keep the bowels regulated with the following :

Mercurial Pill, 1 grain; Ipecac Powder, ½ grain; Compound Rhubarb Pill, 3 grains. *Mix*—for a pill to be taken every night.

Or one ounce of Hiera Picra, or powdered Aloes with Castella, mixed in a pint of gin, which should stand for four or five days, after which a tablespoonful in a glass of water may be taken every morning, or second morning as the case may be.

If the patient is large and fleshy, of full habit, the following is recommended:

Sulphate of Magnesia, 1½ ounce; Compound Infusion of Roses, 5 ounces; Cinnamon Water, 1 ounce. *Mix.*—Dose, two tablespoonfuls once a day.

If there are nervous symptoms prominent, give:

Valerianate of Zinc, 8 grains; Tincture of Valerian, 2 drachms; Orange Flower Water, 3½ ounces; Syrup of Red Poppies, 2 drachms. *Mix.*—Dose, a tablespoonful every six hours.

FALLING OF THE WOMB—(*Prolapsus Uteri.*)

Falling of the womb is simply a sinking down of the organ, and may be so slight as not to be noticed, or so great that the organ will protrude between the legs through the external opening. It is not a disease of the womb itself; but of some of its supports.

So long as the vagina retains its natural size, and the ligaments are but two and a half inches long, the organ will not be displaced. Whatever tends to relax and weaken the system, may cause the complaint. The muscles of the abdomen which support the intestines being weakened from any cause, will allow the intestines to press down upon the womb and its ligaments, and, in consequence of this constant pressure, they give way. Another cause is too early exercise after child-bearing. Flooding, and leucorrhœa or whites, if allowed to continue for a long time will produce it. In delicate females, continued running up and down stairs, also tight lacing, dancing, leaping, and running, particularly during the period of menstruation, when the womb is increased in weight by the blood contained in it. The use of medicines to loosen the bowels, which is very common among many, is still another cause of the disorder.

Most females who are troubled with falling of the womb, think that it is necessary to a cure that they should wear some kind of a support to the abdomen. These supporters, however, do a vast amount of harm, for by being worn tightly around the abdomen, they increase the pressure on the bowels, thus forcing down, more and more, the womb and its appendages. All that is necessary is to raise up the womb to its natural position, and use an instrument that will keep it in place. This instrument is called a pessary. This pessary is a ring, or hollow, cup-shaped globe, made of gold, silver, ivory, wood or gutta percha, and is placed in the vagina, or birth place, thus supporting the womb. The cold hip bath should be used once a day, at the same time injecting cold water into the vagina, with a syringe. Lie down as much as possible, and avoid becoming fatigued. Apply cold bandages to the abdomen, on going to bed.

If the womb has descended to the external orifice, it is often necessary to restore it to its natural position by pressing it upward and backward by a finger or two pressed into the vagina. If the process be accompanied with pain, the vagina should be well washed by injections of thick flax-seed or slippery-elm bark tea for a day or two before the astringent washes are used.

Avoid tight corsets and heavy skirts, suspend the under garments from the shoulders and not from the waist, as is usually done. Use plain vegetable diet and avoid tea, coffee, spirituous drinks and all sensual indulgences. Allow the clothes

to be loose.   These things must be attended to closely.   The diet
should be plain and nourishing, but not stimulating.

. Use an injection of an infusion of White Oak Bark, Geranium,
or a solution of Alum, in the proportion of one ounce to the pint
of water.   If there is inflammation of the womb, this must be
subdued before using the pessary.   Give Tincture of Aconite,
compound powder of Ipecac and Opium, with injections of an infusion of Hops and Lobelia, or an infusion of Belladonna.

If there is heat and difficulty in passing water, drink an infusion of Marsh mallow and Spearmint.   If the patient is weak,
give the following tonic:

Sulphate Quinine, 25 grains; Citrate of Iron, (soluble) 35 grains. Make
into twenty-four powders. Take a powder three times a day, after each meal
in sweet wine.

LEUCORRHŒA—WHITES—FLUOR ALBUS.

The word leucorrhœa is derived from two Greek words, and
means literally a "white discharge."   It is also known as "Fluor
Albus," "Whites," and "Female Weakness," and consists of a
"light colorless discharge from the genital organs, varying in hue
from a whitish or colorless, to a yellowish, light green, or to a
slightly red or brownish; varying in consistency from a thin watery, to a thick, tenacious, ropy substance; and in quantity from
a slight increase in the healthy secretion, to several ounces, in the
twenty-four hours."   This discharge generally occurs between the
age of fifteen and forty-five, seldom during infancy or old age.
When it occurs in young female children, it will not unfrequently
be produced by the presence of pin worms in the vagina, which
make their way there from the rectum.   There will be intense
itching of the parts, and the worms can be removed with a small
piece of cloth, after separating the lips.

This disease may be either acute or chronic.   The acute form
generally results from taking cold, and is simply a catarrhal inflammation of the mucous membrane lining the vagina.   The
chronic form is but a continuation of the acute, and is generally
caused by the acute stage having been neglected or improperly
treated.   Ulceration of the neck of the womb sometimes results.
There are two forms of leucorrhœa:—vaginal leucorrhœa, when
the discharge comes from the walls of the vagina; and cervical
leucorrhœa, when the discharge proceeds from the neck of the
womb.

Causes:—Taking cold from sitting on the ground, or exposure
of the neck and shoulders; over sexual excitement, and sexual intercourse: tight lacing; piles; miscarriages and abortions; dis-
placements of the womb ; purgatives ; improper articles of diet ;
warm injections, or injections of any kind; late hours, etc.   It
may also be hereditary.

The treatment, to be successful, requires that the patient should
first be placed in a favorable condition.   Anything which tends
to excite the disease, must be avoided, as dissipations, late suppers,

etc. The diet must be plain and nourishing, without being stimulating, and be taken regularly. Exercise, short of fatigue, will be beneficial. The clothing should be warm, and worn loosely, especially about the waist. Water is of great importance in the treatment of this trouble. The sitting bath may be used every day, and injections of cold or tepid water should be used, three or four times a day, according to the severity of the discharge.

An injection of weak green tea will be found good in some mild cases, as also sweet cider, a weak solution of alum.

One of the best tonics is the Muriated Tincture of Iron, of which take twenty or twenty-five drops, in half a tumbler of water, three or four times a day. An excellent injection is made by taking three drachms of Tannic acid, and an ounce of Alum, dissolving in a quart of water, and inject one-third, three times a day. The bowels should be kept open by Rochelle or Epsom Salts, or Seidlitz Powder. Where there is great debility of the organs, or when the disease has been brought on by exposure to cold, pregnancy, abortions, etc., the following will be found very successful:

Tincture of Aloes, 2 ounces; Muriated Tincture of Iron, 4 drachms. *Mix.* —Dose, thirty-five drops in water, three times a day.

At the same time use the following injection :

Sulphate of Zinc, (white Vitriol,) 2 drachms; Sugar of Lead, 2 drachms. *Mix* in one quart of water, and use one-fourth for each injection.

www.ingramcontent.com/pod-product-compliance
Lightning Source LLC
Chambersburg PA
CBHW021932190326
41519CB00009B/999